# PULMONARY INFECTION

Edited by **Amer Amal**

**Pulmonary Infection**
Edited by Amer Amal

**Published by InTech**
Janeza Trdine 9, 51000 Rijeka, Croatia



**Publishing Process Manager** Molly Kaliman

**Technical Editor** Teodora Smiljanic

**Cover Designer** InTech Design Team

Additional hard copies can be obtained from orders@intechopen.com

Pulmonary Infection, Edited by Amer Amal
p. cm.
ISBN 978-953-51-0286-1

For EU product safety concerns:
IN TECH d.o.o., Prolaz Marije Krucifikse Kozulić 3, 51000 Rijeka, Croatia,
info@intechopen.com or visit our website at intechopen.com.

# Meet the editor

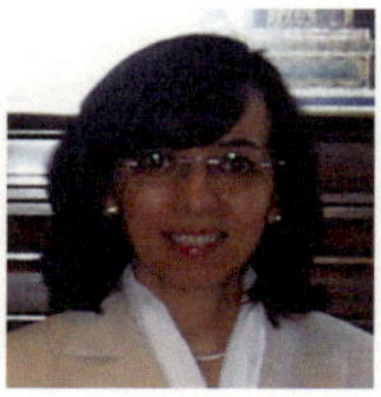

Dr Amer is currently an Assistant Professor at The Ohio State University. She is a faculty in the Department of Microbial Infection and Immunity and the Department of Internal Medicine, Pulmonary Division. Dr Amer is also a member in the Center for Microbial Interface Biology. Her MD and PhD training allowed her to contribute with her knowledge in several developing countries. She trained several undergraduate and graduate students as well as post-doctoral candidates and medical fellows from different parts of the world. Dr Amer's work is focused on the innate immune response to pulmonary pathogens such as Legionella pneumophila and Burkholderia cenocepacia. Legionella targets the elderly and immuno-compromised while Burkholderia targets patients with cystic fibrosis. Dr Amer was among the first to establish the ligands for several NOD-like receptors and their role in inflammation. Dr Amer also explored the role of autophagy as an innate immune response to Legionella and Burkholderia. Her recent work with Burkholderia offers new drug targets for the control of infection with Burkholderia which is resistant to most antibiotics. Dr Amer's long standing studies on the role of caspases during intracellular infection allowed the discovery of novel non-apoptotic functions of caspases.

# Contents

# Preface

Clinical symptoms imply the ubiquity of respiratory infections, however pathogenesis and hence management maybe unique. The aim of this book is to present the recent findings in the pathogenesis of infectious respiratory diseases. Certain chapters depict a quick overview of respiratory infections caused by bacteria, viruses and fungi. Several chapters describe modes of infection, clinical symptoms, diagnosis and treatments for different respiratory infections. Special emphasis was given to tuberculous and non-tuberculous mycobacterial infections in a number of chapters. The insight brought forth from this book can be valuable for both clinicians and scientists.

**Asst. Prof. Dr. Amal Amer, MD, PhD**
Division of Pulmonary, Allergy, Critical Care and Sleep Medicine,
Center for Microbial Interface Biology and The Department of Internal Medicine,
Ohio State University, Columbus Ohio
USA

1

# Latent Tuberculosis: Advances in Diagnosis and Treatment

Dimitrios Basoulis, Georgia Vrioni, Violetta Kapsimali,
Aristeidis Vaiopoulos and Athanasios Tsakris
*Medical School of the National and Kapodistrian University of Athens*
*Greece*

## 1. Introduction

Tuberculosis (TB) is one of the oldest diseases known to affect humans. It is caused by bacteria belonging to the *Mycobacterium tuberculosis* complex and strains of these bacteria have been found in human bones dated from the Neolithic era. It was known to the ancient Greeks, Indians and the Inca, making it a disease with a global distribution even from ancient times. Latent tuberculosis infection refers to a time period where the host has been exposed and infected by the bacteria yet does not exhibit any signs or symptoms of infection. It is estimated that one third of the world, almost 2 billion people suffer from latent tuberculosis infection.

## 2. Epidemiology

Tuberculosis is a multisystemic infection with myriad presentations and manifestations. According to the World Health Organization (WHO) it is estimated that one third of the world's population is currently infected by the bacillus and out of those people 5-10% will exhibit symptoms at some point during their life. WHO estimates that the largest number of new TB cases in 2008 occurred in the South-East Asia Region, which accounted for 35% of incident cases globally. However, the estimated incidence rate in sub-Saharan Africa is nearly twice that of the South-East Asia Region with over 350 cases per 100 000 population (WHO, 2011). Tuberculosis remains the most common cause of infectious disease related mortality worldwide. It is evident by this alone that latent tuberculosis is a serious public health problem, not only due to the possibility of the patients themselves eventually developing active tuberculosis, but also because of the public health risk that they impose.

*M. tuberculosis* is most commonly transmitted from a patient with infectious pulmonary tuberculosis via droplet nuclei, aerosolised by coughing, sneezing or even speaking. The tiny droplets dry rapidly, but the smallest of them (<10μm in diameter) can remain suspended in the atmosphere for several hours. When inhaled, these droplets can reach the terminal airspaces of the lung. Risk factors for transmission include the proximity of contact, the duration of contact, the degree of infectiousness of the case and the shared environment of the contact. It needs to be noted that patients that have sputum smear negative and culture positive tuberculosis are less infectious, whereas patients with culture negative sputum pose essentially no risk for transmission. It is estimated that up to 20 people can be infected by a single patient before tuberculosis can be identified in high prevalence countries. Transmission is more common in tightly packed populations (i.e. overpopulated areas, military personnel etc.) in countries with a higher incidence.

It has been demonstrated that large clusters of TB are associated with an increased number of tuberculin skin test-positive contacts, even after adjusting for other risk factors for transmission. The number of positive contacts was significantly lower for cases with isoniazid-resistant TB compared with cases with fully-susceptible TB. This result has been interpreted to imply some connection between isoniazid resistance and mycobacterial virulence (Verhagen et al., 2011).

After exposure to the bacteria, the patient has a 5-10% chance of developing active tuberculosis. Risk factors that determine this progression include age, the individual's innate susceptibility to disease and level of function of cell-mediated immunity. Clinical illness directly following infection is classified as **primary tuberculosis** and is more common in children. The majority of patients infected will develop disease within a year while the rest will develop latent tuberculosis. Activation of tuberculosis bacilli at any point thereafter is termed **secondary tuberculosis**. Several diseases predispose the patient to develop active tuberculosis with chief amongst them HIV co-infection. It is estimated that nearly all of infected individuals that are HIV positive will at some point develop active tuberculosis; this risk depends on the level of immunosuppression and the CD4+ cell count of the infected patient. Patients with diabetes have 2-5 times increased risk for developing active disease, whereas the relative risk for patients with chronic renal failure climbs to 10-25.

## 3. Pathophysiology of tuberculosis infection

Two models for the pathophysiology of tuberculosis infection and the formation of granulomas have been suggested. The first one is the static model and it is considered to be the traditional one. The second was suggested a few years ago and it is the dynamic model of infection.

### 3.1 The static model

Mycobacteria belong to the family Mycobacteriaceae and the order Actinomycetales. The most important member of the *Mycobacterium tuberculosis* complex is the namesake organism, *Mycobacterium tuberculosis.* The complex also includes *M. bovis* (the bovine tubercle bacillus), *M. africanum* (isolated from cases in West, Central and East Africa), *M. microti* (a less virulent rarer bacillus), *M. pinnipedii* and *M. canettii* (very rare isolates). *M. tuberculosis* is a slow-growing, obligate aerobe and obligate pathogen. Most often, it is neutral on Gram's staining, however, once stained, the bacilli cannot be de-colorised by acid alcohol, hence the characterization as acid-fast and the reason they are best seen using the Ziehl-Neelsen stain. This ability of mycobacteria is derived from the high content of mycolic acids, long chain fatty acids and other lipids found in abundance in the cell wall of mycobacteria (Harada, 1976; Harada et al, 1977). In the mycobacterial cell wall, lipids are linked to underlying arabinolactan and peptidoglycan, which confers a high resistance to antibiotics due to low permeability of this structure. Another element of the cell wall structure is the lipoarabinomannan which is crucial to the mycobacterium's survival within the host's macrophages. All of these proteins, characteristic of *M. tuberculosis* are included in the purified protein derivative (PPD, a precipitate of non-species-specific antigens obtained from filtrates of heat-sterilised, concentrated broth cultures.

The majority of inhaled bacilli are trapped at the level of the upper airways and expelled. A small fraction (<10%) will descend further down the bronchial tree. When the inhaled droplet nuclei reach the terminal airspaces of the lung, the bacilli, transported with the droplets, begin to grow for 2-12 weeks before any immune response from the host can be elicited. The host's immune system responds when the bacillary load reaches 1000-10,000 cells. Non-specifically activated alveolar macrophages will eventually begin to ingest the bacilli and sequester them from the host.

Phagocytes have 2 methods of dealing with the mycobacteria. Fusing the phagosomes containing the mycobacteria with lysosomes they create phagolysosomes. Phagolysosomes are the product of a fusion-fission process between the lysosomes, the phagosomes and other intracellular vesicles. The $Ca^{+2}$ signalling pathway and recruitment of vacuolar-proton transporting ATPase (vH+-ATPase) lead to a decrease in the pH of the phagolysosome, that in turn allows acid hydrolases to function efficiently for their microbicidal effect. Another way that phagocytes deal with the mycobacteria is through ubiquitination of mycobacterial cell wall and membrane components, which in turn leads to increased susceptibility to nitric oxide produced by the phagocytes. This process leads to phagocyte apoptosis (Beisiegel et al 2009; Bermudez & Goodman, 1996; Chan & Flynn, 2004; Cooper, 2009; Pieters, 2008; Ahmad, 2010).

This form of defence, however, proves inefficient as the bacilli have the ability to survive inside the macrophages by modulating the behaviour of its phagosome, preventing its fusion with acidic, hydrolytically-active lysosomes (Pieters, 2008; Russel et al 2009) The escape of *M. tuberculosis* from macrophage destruction is dependent on the 6-kDa early secreted antigenic target (ESAT-6) protein and ESX-1 protein secretion system encoded by the region of difference 1 (RD1). The ESAT-6 protein associates with liposomes containing dimyristoylphosphatidylcholine and cholesterol and causes destabilization and lysis of liposomes. It can also infiltrate the phagosome's membrane and cause lysis of the phagosome, enabling the mycobacteria to escape (Brodin et al, 2004; de Jonge et al, 2007; Derrick & Morris, 2007; Kinhikar et al, 2010).

In this initial stage of interaction, either the macrophages manage to contain the bacillary reproduction through sequestration and production of cytokines and proteolytic enzymes, or the bacilli manage to survive and multiply, leading to macrophage lysis. Through chemotaxis, monocytes arrive at the site of infection to ingest the bacilli after the macrophage lysis. Either through lysis or apoptosis the mycobacterial antigens are exposed and presented to T lymphocytes that will carry out the burden of the host's immune response orchestration.

Following these events, the host's immune system activates two more mechanisms to battle the invading bacteria: a **tissue damaging response** and a **macrophage activating response**. The tissue damaging response is a delayed-type hypersensitivity reaction to bacillary antigens leading to the destruction of "infected" macrophages. The macrophage activation focuses on activating specific macrophages to ingest and destroy the bacteria. Local macrophages are activated when the non-specific macrophages present bacillary antigens to

T lymphocytes, stimulating them to release lymphokines. Depending on which one of the two mechanisms is predominant, the subsequent form of tuberculosis is determined.

If the macrophage activation predominates, large numbers of activated macrophages arrive at the site of infection and granulomatous lesions begin to form. During this early stage and under the influence of a vascular endothelial growth factor (VEGF), the granuloma becomes highly vascularised which in turn will provide the pathway for the lymphocytes and macrophages to arrive at the site (Alatas F et al, 2004) Once there, the macrophages will further differentiate into different cells such as multi-nucleated giant cells, epitheliod cells and foamy macrophages. These cells will form the outer wall of the granuloma, now dubbed tubercle. The structure becomes much more stratified and a fibrous cuff forms outside the macrophage layer. Lymphocytes move away from the centre and aggregate outside this fibrous layer (Cáceres et al 2009).

The tissue damaging response on the other hand leads to destruction of macrophages that fail to contain the bacilli and in turn creates a necrotic area at the centre of the tubercle with dead macrophages. Due to low oxygen, presence of nitric oxide, nutrient deficiency and very acidic pH the mycobacteria cannot continue to multiply inside the tubercle centres, yet they can survive and remain dormant (Ahmad, 2010; Ohno et al, 2003; Voskuil et al, 2003). The central necrotic region resembles cheese in texture and has granted the name caseous necrosis to this process. At this point, some of the tubercles calcify and heal while others evolve further.

Two distinct types of granulomas have been identified. The classic caseous granulomas are composed of epithelial macrophages, neutrophils, and other immune cells surrounded by fibroblasts. *M. tuberculosis* resides inside macrophages in the central caseous necrotic region. The second type of granulomas (fibrotic lesions) is composed of mainly fibroblasts and contains very few macrophages. The exact location of viable *M. tuberculosis* in these lesions is not known (Barry et al, 2009). It needs to be noted that even the healed, fibrotic tubercles can still contain mycobacteria in a dormant state.

It has been suggested that the caseating centre of the granuloma is not the site where the host's immune response is organized and maintained, but rather that site is at the outer layers of the tubercle, where the macrophages can present their antigens to the lymphocytic population of the tubercle. This formation resembles a secondary lymphoid organ and is theorised to be better suited to orchestrate the host's immune response, as suggested by the high proliferative activity only observed in peripheral follicle-like structures (Ulrichs et al, 2004).

If the tissue damaging response predominates, due to a week response from the macrophages, the initial lesion cannot be contained and continues to grow at the expense of the surrounding tissue. Bronchial walls and blood vessels are destroyed in this process (hence why haemoptysis is a chief symptom in rampant tuberculosis) and cavities are gradually formed (Zvi et al, 2008).

The mycobacterial cell wall components are recognized by host receptors that include toll-like receptors (TLRs), nucleotide-binding oligomerisation domain (NOD)-like receptors (NLRs), and C-type lectins, including mannose receptor (MR), the dendritic cell-specific intercellular adhesion molecule grabbing nonintegrin (DC-SIGN), macrophage inducible C-type lectin (Mincle) and dendritic cell-associated C-type lectin-1 (Dectin-1). The TLR signalling is the main arm of the innate immune response and *M. tuberculosis* phagocyted through different receptors may have a different fate (Harding & Boom, 2010; Ishikawa E et al, 2009; Jo, 2008; Jo et al, 2007; Noss et al, 2001).

Cell mediated immunity, more specifically macrophages and CD4+ T lymphocytes, plays a very important role in the above process. The infected macrophages produce a host of cytokines: Interleukin 1 (IL1) which leads to the development of fever, interleukin 6 (IL6) which leads to hyperglobulinemia and tumour necrosis factor α (TNF-α) that contributes to the killing of mycobacteria, the formation of caseating granulomas, fever and weight loss. As mentioned earlier, non-specific macrophages are also responsible for presenting the bacillary antigens to the T cells and eliciting their response (Khader & Cooper, 2008; Kursar et al 2007). Activated T helper Type 1 lymphocytes participate in the destruction of infected cells through an MHC class II restricted process. They also produce interferon γ (IFN-γ) and interleukin 2 (IL2) and promote cell-mediated immunity. Once the bacillary growth is stabilized, the presence of CD8+ T cells appears to gain importance, both for the production of IFN-γ and an increase in the cytotoxic activity. This is a period of stalemate where the bacillary load remains relatively constant and the infection is in a state of latency (Bodnar et al, 2001; Russel et al, 2009).

More recently, it was demonstrated that IL1-beta, a subset of interleukin 1, which plays an important part as mediator in the host's immune response, is induced when ESAT-6 is secreted from the bacilli. IL1-beta is activated through the inflammasome, a caspase activating protein complex. Caspases are cysteine-aspartic proteases that play a part in inflammation response and apoptosis. Mycobacteria have developed the ability to halt the inflammasome's formation by secreting a $Zn^{+2}$ metalloprotease, encoded by the zmp1 gene. Mycobacteria genetically modified for zmp1 deletion and through the secretion of ESAT-6 lead to IL1-beta activation and elicit a stronger immune response from the host leading to improved mycobacterial clearance by macrophages, and lower bacterial burden in the lungs of aerosol-infected mice (Danelishvili, 2010; Lalor, 2011; Master 2008; Mishra, 2010). Mycobacteria secrete their own enzymes (Rv3654c and Rv3655c) within the macrophage cytoplasm with the ability to cleave caspase-8. In this manner, the bacilli prevent macrophage apoptosis by preventing the inflammasome's formation and promote cellular lysis (Danelishvili, 2010). It has been demonstrated that it is more beneficial to bacterial growth if the macrophages are steered towards lysis as opposed to apoptosis. Necrosis was correlated with Caspase 3 activity and bacterial growth, whereas activation of calcium, TNF-alpha and Caspase 8 was associated with apoptosis and decreased bacterial load (Arcila et al, 2007).

Humoral immunity seems to play a much lesser role if any. The evidence that B-cells and M. tuberculosis-specific antibodies can mediate protection against extracellular *M. tuberculosis* is highly controversial as their contribution is probably of minor importance (TBNET, 2009).

The host's immune response can eventually cause more problems through tissue destruction and uncontrolled activation of macrophages and lymphocytes. For this reason there is a negative feedback mechanism in place, to control the extent of the response. A family of receptor tyrosine kinases provide this negative feedback mechanism to both, TLR-mediated and cytokine-driven proinflammatory immune responses (Liew, 2005). Again, the mycobacteria have developed mechanisms to take advantage of this process in order to halt the immune response to their benefit. Several *M. tuberculosis* cell wall components or protein products such as 19-kDa lipoprotein, glycolipids (particularly Man-LAM), trehalose dimycolate (cord factor) can modulate antigen-processing pathways by MHC class I, MHC class II and CD1 molecules, phagolysosome formation and other macrophage intracellular signalling pathways (Ahmad, 2010; Bowdish et al, 2009; Gehring et al, 2004; Harding & Boom, 2010; Jo et al, 2007; Nigou et al, 2001; Noss et al, 2001; Pecora et al; 2006). This results in a subset of macrophages that are unable to present mycobacterial antigens to T lymphocytes

It is hypothesized that the infection sustains itself not through replicating bacilli forming equilibrium with those being destroyed by the host's immune system, but through a population of non-replicating bacilli that can withstand the immune response. The evidence to this is indirect, suggested by the lack of cellular debris in the granuloma centres of infected mice (Rees & Hart, 1961). It is believed that the host's immune response is driven by antigens produced during active multiplication of the bacilli and thus, those that remain dormant would not sustain that response to its maximum potential (Andersen, 1997).

### 3.2 The dynamic model

More recently a dynamic model of infection was proposed able to give some logical explanations to some short-comings of the static model. The first question posed was how it is possible for the mycobacteria to remain dormant in the tubercle environment when the host is trying to re-structure the damaged tissues. The alveolar macrophages have a lifespan of 3 months, yet according to the static model, they exist in stalemate with the mycobacteria for a much longer period of time, whether as part of the middle layer of the granuloma or as part of the caseous centre having phagocyted bacilli and sustaining them in their dormant state (Cardona, 2009).

The second question was how did the bacilli reactivate themselves from their dormant state, as it has been demonstrated that the resuscitation factors necessary for this are only produced by active bacilli (Cardona, 2009; Shleeva et al, 2002).

The third question posed seeks an explanation based on a physiological model regarding the ability of isoniazid to treat latent tuberculosis when it is known that isoniazid can only take effect on actively multiplying bacilli (Cardona, 2009; TBNET, 2009).

According to the dynamic model that has been suggested, the granulomas are not static formations but rather, inside the granuloma, there exists a balance between inactive dormant bacilli, rapidly multiplicating ones, dying bacilli and cellular debris constantly being removed from the site (TBNET, 2009). The exact nature of the metabolic state of mycobacteria within the macrophages in the granuloma is a matter of great debate and investigation.

The size of the actively multiplicating mycobacterial load in the granuloma determines the antigen-specific re-stimulation of memory T lymphocytes. On the other hand, if the mycobacteria are mostly contained within macrophages in their dormant state, it is more likely that T cell immunity will begin to decline. This in turn would explain why a tuberculin skin test can revert to negative after exposure at a rate of about 5% per year (TBNET, 2009).

Perhaps the most important element in this proposed model is the role of the foamy cell, i.e. alveolar macrophages at the end of their life cycle and filled with lipids, due to phagocytosis of extracellular debris, mostly consisting of lipid-rich cellular membrane remains. The mycobacteria phagocyted by these cells can survive through the mechanisms explained earlier. The dynamic model suggests that the mycobacteria can continue to grow albeit at very slow rates instead of becoming dormant. The slower metabolic rate provides resistance to stress and reduces the nutritional needs of the bacilli, thus allowing their survival (Cardona, 2009; Muñoz-Elias et al, 2005). It has not been fully researched but evidence suggests that mycobacteria can escape the phagosomes of the foamy cells and reach the bronchial tree and become aerosolised.

Foamy cells provide a stressful environment that conditions the bacilli to become more resistant. This in turn, confers them the ability to better survive in the open air and according to some studies explains why they are more virulent. Moreover, the high lipid content of the foamy cells also provides triglycerides to the bacilli that will in turn provide them with nutrients in new infection sites in the event of starvation. In fact the highly aggressive Beijing strains have also been found to contain large amounts of lipids, which would at least partly account for the greater virulence (Garton et al, 2002; Neyrolles et al, 2006; Peyron et al, 2008). Finally the high lipid content of foamy cells when exposed to the alveolar spaces will contribute to increased surfactant concentration and thus will make aerosolisation of the bacteria easier (Cardona, 2009).

Growing bacteria are easy to combat since they cannot survive in stressful environments. The dynamic model offers a different explanation of the mechanism, with which the host's immune system focuses on the non-replicating bacteria. The phagocyted bacilli, as explained in the static model, will eventually lead to lysis or apoptosis of the macrophages. This cellular debris and the extracellular bacteria will form the population of the non-replicating bacteria at the caseous centre. The attraction of specific macrophages and neutrophils will provide a new breeding ground for the active bacteria and also material for the formation of the foamy cells, as they will phagocyte cellular membrane remnants to clear the debris from the caseous centre of the granuloma. The bacilli, inside the foamy cells, under these circumstances, will eventually find themselves within the bronchial spaces and after they are aerosolised they will reinfect the host at new sites. Due to their higher virulence they will manage to overcome the initial immune response and form a new granuloma to repeat the same sequence of events (Cardona, 2009). At the new site of infection the bacilli are actively multiplying again and thus are susceptible to isoniazid. This would explain why a single-drug nine month treatment is effective in most cases of latent tuberculosis.

## 4. Latent tuberculosis and reactivation

Mycobacteria are completely eradicated only in about 10% of the cases, while in the remaining, the bacilli survive for years to come, through the processes explained. This state has been termed **latent tuberculosis infection.** In any event where the host's immune response dwindles, there is a risk for the bacilli to reactivate themselves and lead to active tuberculosis infection. Most of the new cases of tuberculosis in low incidence countries are the result of such reactivation of latent tuberculosis infections. It is of interest to note that expression of DosR-regulated dormancy antigens continues even in this latent stage of infection, providing a promising new target for vaccines that would help battle latent TB infections in the future (Leyten et al, 2006; Lin & Ottenhoff, 2008). It is also probable that *M. tuberculosis*, during the latent stage of infection can form spore-like structures, typically seen with other mycobacteria, in response to prolonged stationary phase or nutrient starvation, for its survival (Ghosh et al, 2009).

The reactivation of latent infection requires *M. tuberculosis* to exit dormancy. This is mainly achieved through the effects of a family of five proteins, dubbed resuscitation promoting factors (Rpfs), that have the effect of a lytic transglycosylase. These molecules were found to be able to cause degradation to cell wall components of the mycobacteria. It is not exactly known how this activity relates to the resuscitation process, it is however theorised that the end result of this enzymatic activity is changes to the mycobacterial cell-wall, overcoming the environmental restraints to the bacterial multiplication. Another theory states that the changes brought to the cell wall, lead to production and secretion of peptidoglycans with the ability to modulate the environment and the host's immune response (Hett et al, 2007; Tufariello et al, 2006). It needs be noted that *M. tuberculosis* bacilli found in the sputum of patients with latent infection and after deletion of the Rpfs encoding genes, can only be cultured when Rpfs are introduced to the growth material and thus resuscitation is possible (Mukamolova et al, 2010), however for non-dormant mycobacteria it seems that the Rpfs are not important for their multiplication (Kana et al, 2008).

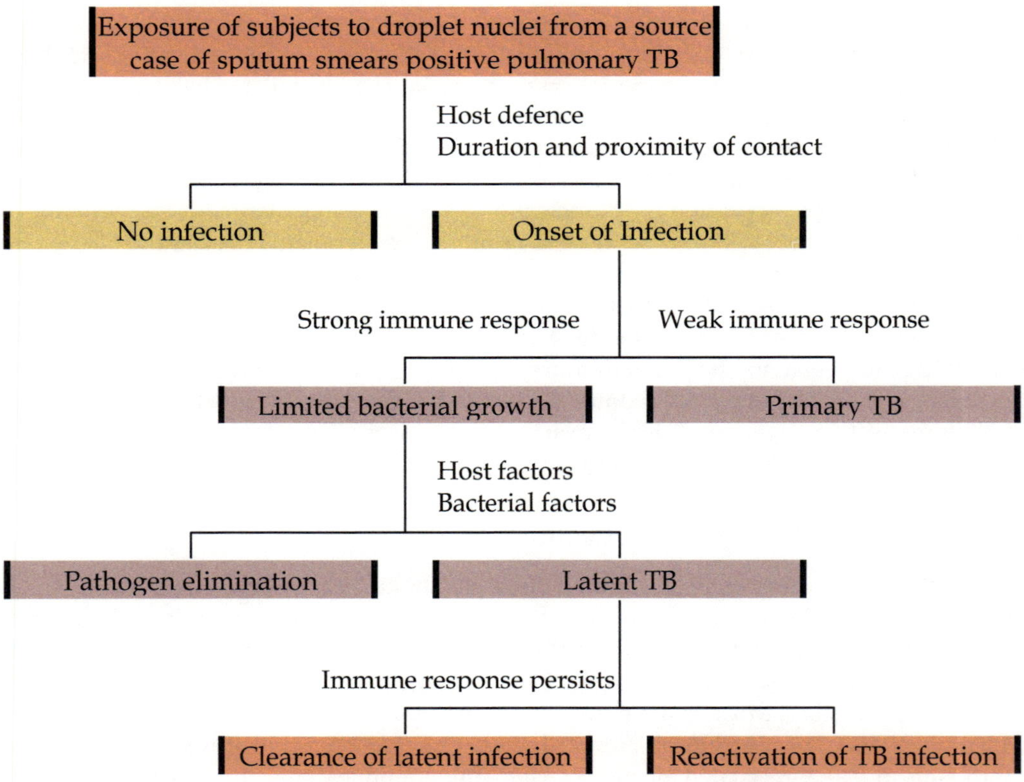


Fig. 1. Natural progression of tuberculosis, adapted from Ahmad, 2010

It has also been demonstrated that amongst the Rpfs, those that seem to be the most important are RpfA and RpfB. Infected mice with strains of mycobacteria with deletion of the genes encoding these specific Rpfs, were found to be more resistant to TB reactivation and also their macrophages were found to produce larger quantities of TNF-α and IL6 (Russel-Goldman et al, 2008). These resuscitation factors are another possible target for future vaccines against latent TB (Zvi et al, 2008).

## 5. Latent tuberculosis diagnosis

Diagnosis of latent tuberculosis is a matter of active current research due to the difficulties presented in identifying patients with latent infection. There is no question that controlling contacts and identifying people who are carrying the bacilli would be the best prevention plan. However, due to the lack of any physical signs or symptoms and the fact that all or most of the bacilli during this state remain dormant, it is very difficult to elicit an immune system response that would be evident to the observer. This in turn means that it is difficult to identify individuals with latent infection. An ideal test for latent tuberculosis infection diagnosis should meet the following criteria:

- High sensitivity in all populations at risk.
- High specificity regardless of BCG vaccination and infection with environmental mycobacteria.
- Reliability and stability over time.
- Objective criteria for positive result, affordability and easy administration.
- Ability to distinguish recently infected individuals with increased risk of progression to active tuberculosis.

There are currently two groups of tests for latent tuberculosis infection diagnosis: tuberculin skin tests (TST) and interferon-γ release assays (IGRA).

### 5.1 The tuberculin skin test

Historically, the most accurate method for detecting if an individual had come in contact with *M. tuberculosis* was the tuberculin skin test (TST). This test measures the hosts' *in vivo* immune response in the form of a cell-mediated delayed hypersensitivity reaction to a mixture of more than 200 *M. tuberculosis* antigens, termed as purified protein derivative (PPD). The PPD is a crude mixture of antigens, not specific to *M.* tuberculosis, but also found in other mycobacteria such as the BCG bacillus, *M.* bovis and even non-tuberculous mycobacteria. This mixture is intradermally injected, usually at the inner side of the forearm and the test result is read as an induration on the site of injection after 48-72 hours (Huebner et al 1993). This reaction may last for up to 1 month, depending on the quality and quantity of the initial reaction. Strong reactions may result in tissue necrosis, which is the only absolute contraindication to the TST (TBNET, 2009). The induration is caused due to the introduction of the antigens that causes non-specific neutrophils and antigen-specific T lymphocytes to arrive at the site and sparkle an inflammatory cascade of cytokine production. The migration of immune cells to the site seems to have a biphasic distribution: an initial nonspecific infiltration where the neutrophils arrive at the site, taking place in the first 4-6 hours and which is an event that also occurs in nonsensitised subjects and a second specific peak, where the specific T cells arrive at the site (Kenney et al, 1987; Platt et al, 1983;

Poulter et al, 1982; TBNET, 2009). The lymphocyte population is a mix of CD4+ and CD8+ cells with the former being always greater in number (Gibbs et al, 1984). The lymphocytic infiltration is at first perivascular and under the influence of early cytokines, such as IFN-γ, TNF-α and TNF-β, the endothelium is stimulating into expressing adhesion molecules (E-selectin), increasing the permeability of the vascular walls and enabling the cells to migrate to the dermis. Regulatory T-cells influence the size of the induration of the tuberculin skin test. Cutaneous CD4 T-cells accumulating after tuberculin PPD stimulation in the skin are predominantly of a CD45 RO memory phenotype (Sarrazin et al, 2009). The criteria for the test's interpretation vary considerably and depend on the nature of the population being tested. They are arbitrary and the result of international consensus.

In the United States, according to the Center for Disease Control (CDC), 5 tuberculin units (TUs) are used and a test is considered positive for the general population with no known TB contacts when the induration measures 15mm or more. An induration of 10 or more millimetres is considered positive in recent immigrants (< 5 years) from high-prevalence countries, injection drug users, residents and employees of high-risk congregate settings, mycobacteriology laboratory personnel, persons with clinical conditions that place them at high risk, children < 4 years of age, infants, children, and adolescents exposed to adults in high-risk categories. Finally, an induration of 5 or more millimetres is considered positive in HIV-infected persons, a recent contact of a person with TB disease, persons with fibrotic changes on chest radiograph consistent with prior TB, patients with organ transplants, persons who are immunosuppressed for other reasons (e.g., taking the equivalent of >15 mg/day of prednisone for 1 month or longer, taking TNF-α antagonists, etc.) (CDC, 2011).

In Europe, the situation differs from country to country depending on the incidence and prevalence of TB. In countries with high incidence, such as former Soviet Union countries, a 10mm induration is considered positive. In most European countries 2 TUs are used and interpretation of the results follows the same guidelines as in the US (ECDC, 2011).

As with every screening test, TST has a chance of false positive and false negative results. Possible false positive reactions are caused due to infections with non-tuberculous mycobacteria, previous vaccination with BCG, incorrect method of TST administration (including wrong amount of PPD injected as well as injecting it subcutaneously rather than intradermally), incorrect interpretation of reaction (more often than many would assume, doctors and/or nurses measure the erythema caused by the immune response rather than the induration leading to overestimation of the reaction caused), incorrect bottle of antigen used. False negative results are caused by cutaneous anergy (anergy is the inability to react to skin tests because of a weakened immune system, such as in HIV patients or patients under immunosuppression, particularly those taking anti-TNF-α medications for autoimmune conditions), recent TB infection (within 8-10 weeks of exposure), very old TB infection (many years), very young age (less than 6 months old), recent live-virus vaccination (e.g., measles and smallpox), overwhelming TB disease (tuberculosis by itself is thought to cause a degree of immunosuppression to the host in these advanced cases), some viral illnesses (e.g., measles and chicken pox), incorrect method of TST administration, incorrect interpretation of reaction (ECDC, 2011; CDC, 2011).

Of special consideration is the so-called booster effect after TST testing. In certain people, who have been exposed to *M. tuberculosis*, the ability of their immune system to react to the PPD antigens might have diminished over the course of time. These patients when tested with the TST would have a negative reading. However, reintroducing the tuberculosis antigens to their immune system by the test itself stimulates their immune system to react more fiercely to these antigens. Subsequent tests in these individuals would result as positive even though they haven't been exposed to the bacilli in the time between the two tests. In a sense, the first TST "boosted" the results of the second one. In certain populations, the CDC suggests performing a two-step test in order to identify possible false negative first tests and prevent unnecessary treatment. Such populations include health-care workers, doctors, nurses or nursing home residents, whose status with regards to tuberculosis exposure and/or infection is important to know.

It is evident that the TST has several limitations to its use, which in turn sparked the interest in developing new diagnostic tools such as the IGRAs. Such limitations include a high proportion of false positive and false negative results, difficulty in separating true infection from the effects of BCG vaccination and NTM infection, technical problems in administration, immune response boosting after repeated TST, complicated and subjective interpretation and a need for a second visit for the interpretation of the test's result.

### 5.2 The interferon-γ release assays

Interferon-γ release assay kit tests were developed the past decade as an alternative to the TST. They are whole-blood tests that can aid in diagnosing *M. tuberculosis* infection, including both latent tuberculosis infection and active disease. They are indirect *in vitro, ex vivo* tests that measure the production of interferon-γ by a patient's T lymphocytes after the latter are incubated with specific M. tuberculosis antigens *in vitro* (Andersen et al, 2000; Harboe et al, 1996; Mahairas et al, 1996). To conduct the test, fresh blood sample from the patient is mixed with the antigens and the response is measured either by measuring the produced interferon through enzyme-linked immunosorbent assay (ELISA), rapid enzyme-linked immunospot assay or by measuring the number of activated T cells through flow cytometry. The difference in method used is what distinguishes the two commercially available kits. QuantiFERON-TB Gold In-Tube (QFT-GIT, by Cellestis Limited, Carnegie, Victoria, Australia) uses the ELISA method and the T-SPOT (by Oxford Immunotec Limited, Abingdon, UK) uses the ELISPOT. It is interesting to mention that initially IGRAs would use the PPD as antigen but still follow the same principle and in an interesting twist of fate, it has been suggested to use the specific IGRA antigens for TST, as these antigens have been found to elicit a distinctive immune response with induration on animals. IGRAs are performed on fresh blood specimens.

The antigens used in these methods are peptides derived from ESAT-6, CFP-10 and for the Quantiferon method TB7.7 proteins of the mycobacteria. The first two are encoded at the region of difference (RD) 1 genetic locum whereas the third at the RD11, regions that are deleted from the *M. bovis* BCG genome and are absent in most environmental mycobacteria, with the exception of *M. kansasii, M. szulgai* and *M. marinum* (TBNET, 2009). During earlier stages of the method's development, the entire protein product was used. The early secretory antigenic target (ESAT) is a 6kDa protein and the culture filtrate protein (CFP-10) is a 10kDa protein. Together they form an heterodimeric complex and depend on each other for stability. They are secreted through the ESX1 secretion system and are considered to be an indication of virulence. Their role is not fully understood but they seem to induce lysis through integration on the macrophage cellular membrane (Brodin et al, 2004; de Jonge et al,

2007; Derrick & Morris, 2007; Kinhikar et al, 2010; Renshaw et al, 2005). Even less is known regarding TB7.7. IGRA techniques support the dynamic model for latent TB since they detect IFN-γ produced by T cells, with a short lifespan that have been activated by macrophages that presented to them the tuberculosis antigens (Cardona, 2009).

For the QFT-GIT (Table 1), 1 ml of blood is drawn into one of each of three special testing tubes. These are precoated and heparinised by the manufacturer. Within 16 hours the tubes must be incubated for another 16 to 24 hours at 37 °C. After centrifugation, the plasma is harvested to be further processed. QFT-GIT collection tubes contain a gel plug that separates the plasma from the cells when centrifuged. The plasma can be used immediately or at a later point in time. Results are interpreted according to the manufacturer's recommendations (ECDC, 2011).

| Result | IFN-γ concentration (International Units per ml, IU/ml) | | |
|---|---|---|---|
| | *M. tuberculosis* antigens | Nil | PHA |
| Positive | ≥ 0.35 IU/ml and ≥ 25% over nil | ≤ 8.0 IU/ml | Any |
| Negative | < 0.35 IU/ml or < 25% over nil | ≤ 8.0 IU/ml | ≥ 0.5 IU/ml |
| Indeterminate | < 0.35 IU/ml or < 25% over nil | ≤ 8.0 IU/ml | < 0.5 IU/ml |
| | Any | > 8.0 IU/ml | Any |

Table 1. Quantiferon results interpretation, adapted from ECDC, 2011

For the T-SPOT assay (Table 2), 8 ml of blood are required and the assay must be performed within eight hours of blood collection. Alternatively, the manufacturer also provides a reagent (T-Cell Xtend) which extends processing time to 32 hours after blood collection. The T-cell-containing peripheral blood mononuclear cell fraction is separated from whole blood and distributed to the microtitre plate wells (250,000 cells/well) provided in the assay kit. Following 16 to 20 hours incubation, the number of IFN-γ-secreting T-cells (represented as spot-forming units) can be detected by ELISPOT assay. As with QFT-GIT the test's results are interpreted according to the manufacturer's recommendations (ECDC, 2011).

| Result | Spot count | | | | |
|---|---|---|---|---|---|
| | *M. tuberculosis* antigens | | | Nil | PHA |
| | ESAT-6 | | CFP-10 | | |
| Positive | ≥ 6 over nil | and/or | ≥ 6 over nil | ≤ 10 | Any |
| Negative | ≤ 5 over nil | and/or | ≤ 5 over nil | ≤ 10 | ≥ 20 |
| Borderline | If for any antigen highest is 5 - 7 over nil | | | < 10 | ≥ 20 |
| Indeterminate | ≤ 6 over nil | and | ≤ 6 over nil | ≤ 10 | < 20 |
| | Any | | | > 10 | Any |

Table 2. T-Spot results interpretation, adapted from ECDC, 2011

The presence of negative and positive controls ensures that IGRAs are correctly performed. The three testing tubes contain the mycobacteria antigens (Mtb), no antigens (Nil) and phytohaemagglutinin A (PHA), a T-cell activating mitogen. The Nil vial serves as the negative control for the process whereas the PHA as the positive one. If there is IFN-γ production in the Mtb tube, none in the Nil and any amount in the PHA, it means that the result is a positive one because it would imply that the sample's lymphocytes reacted to the antigens as expected and did not react to any other antigens that might have contaminated the sample. If on the other hand there is no IFN-γ production in the Mtb tube and the Nil tube but there is in the PHA one, it implies that the lymphocytes react normally to the PHA antigen yet they do not react when exposed to the bacilli antigens and therefore these lymphocytes haven't met these antigens before. Finally, the results are indeterminate if at any point there is IFN-γ production in the Nil tube, which might imply contamination or there is increased baseline interferon production or if there is no sufficient production in the PHA tube, which might imply anergy. Technical factors (sample collection, storage and transportation) might also contribute to returning indeterminate results (ECDC, 2011).

There is a lot of debate on whether IGRAs are indeed more reliable than the traditional TST. In Germany, Denmark and Switzerland, IGRAs have substituted TST when screening populations receiving anti-TNF-α therapies. The US, Australia, France and Denmark use either TST or IGRAs, whereas Canada, the United Kingdom, Italy, Spain, Australia and Slovakia to name a few, support a 2-step approach using both TST and IGRAs in an attempt to increase sensitivity and specificity of both methods. The two-step approach seems to be the most favoured strategy for IGRA use, especially in BCG vaccinated contacts.

IGRAs have some distinct advantages over TST with regards to diagnosing latent tuberculosis infection. IGRA testing requires a single patient visit to conduct the test and results can be available within the day. Moreover there is no "booster" effect associated with IGRAs since they are *ex vivo, in vitro* tests. Finally, due to the specificity of the *M. tuberculosis* antigens used, BCG vaccination does not cause false positive results. Due to the positive control, IGRAs are able to differentiate between immunocompromised hosts and negative results with more accuracy. In the TBNET/ECDC systematic review and meta-analysis (Sester et al. 2010) IGRAs were also found to have greater sensitivity in diagnosing active TB infection compared to the TST, 80% for QFT-GIT, 81% for T-Spot compared to only 65% for the TST. In the same review, specificity was found to be 79% (75-82%) for QFT-GIT, 59% (56-62%) for T-spot and 75% (72-78%) for TST. Sensitivity to diagnose latent TB infection was found 67%, 87% and 71% for QFT-GTI, T-Spot and TST respectively, whereas specificity for latent TB infection was 99%, 98% and 88% respectively (Diel et al, 2011; Menzies et al, 2007; Pai et al, 2008; Sester et al, 2010).

Current consensus amongst the European countries is that IGRAs can be included in screening for latent TB infection, albeit there is not enough evidence yet to provide a clear picture. Nonetheless it can provide an extra step in establishing a diagnosis. On the other hand, due to their high negative predictive value for immunocompetent patients, negative IGRA results can safely exclude progression to active disease, albeit it does not rule out the possibility of latent infection (Diel et al, 2011). Applying the IGRAs to specimens from possible infection sites (i.e. Bronchoalveolar Lavage) as opposed to blood samples, especially in immunodeficient individuals can help distinguish between active and latent TB (Jafari et al, 2009). In diagnosing active tuberculosis we mention for completeness, that current consensus is that IGRAs do not have a place in routine screening, yet in certain cases when there is a strong clinical suspicion yet no laboratory proof, they can contribute. Neither IGRAs nor TST can replace the standard laboratory tools for diagnosing active tuberculosis (ECDC, 2011).

As with the TST, IGRAs also have some shortcomings. Perhaps most importantly IGRAs, just like TST are unable to distinguish between latent and active infection when limited to blood testing. Moreover, blood samples need to be processed within 8-30 hours after collection; otherwise the white blood cells will gradually become non-responsive to the antigenic stimulation. Errors in collecting or transporting blood specimens or in running and interpreting the assay can decrease the accuracy of IGRAs. Since these techniques are relatively new, there is still limited data on the use of IGRAs in certain population groups such as children younger than 5 years of age, HIV patients, anti-TNF-α treated patients or in general immunocompromised patients. Finally there is a significant cost to this process as opposed to the fairly cheap TST method.

Finally, another method is being developed for use that employs flow cytometry for the detection of interferon producing lymphocytes. This method is not yet commercially available and due to the high cost of the process it is not known yet if it will contribute to latent tuberculosis diagnosis (Fuhrmann et all 2008). There are experimental methods detecting antibodies against tuberculosis antigens, but as mentioned already humoral immunity plays a small part in tuberculosis if any at all and thus these methods so far have no clinical application (El-Shazly, 2007). Most recently the WHO issued a statement asking countries to ban antibodies based tests for the diagnosis of tuberculosis (WHO, 2011).

## 6. Latent tuberculosis treatment

Individuals with known contacts with patients suffering from active tuberculosis and who test positive with the aforementioned methods are considered, given reasonable clinical suspicion, to have latent infection. They are eligible to receive treatment in order to prevent them from developing an active infection. In some cases (i.e. children, HIV patients) even without TST or IGRAs supporting, clinical suspicion alone is enough to start treatment and re-test the patient at a later time to verify the result of the diagnostic tests. Treatment for latent tuberculosis is less expensive than for active and preventing the disease provides overall a great economic benefit for the health-care system.

Current guidelines (American Thoracic Society & CDC, 2000, revised 2005) in the US, suggest a 9-month daily treatment with isoniazid (INH) 5mg/kg up to 300mg. This can be reduced to only 6 months, for adults seronegative for HIV co-infection. In most cases the 9 month treatment plan is followed since it has been show to achieve better results (70% complete remission vs. 60% for the 6 month regimen). In very few cases a 12-month regimen is recommended, particularly for populations with a higher incidence of active tuberculosis (TBNET, 2009).

As is the problem with most tuberculosis therapies there is a high amount of non-compliant patients contributing to failure of treatment. One solution would be to enforce Directly Observed Treatment (DOT) for patients taking isoniazid for latent tuberculosis, but such a decision comes with a high financial cost. Under these circumstances, treatment can be modified to a 2/week regimen at a dose of 15mg/kg up to 900mg. Isoniazid side-effects include polyneuropathy, preventable with administration of B6 vitamin and hepatic toxicity that remains a prime reason for discontinuation of treatment. Studies have shown that 10-20% of patients will have an increase in liver transaminases and about 2% will have clinically significant hepatitis, with that percentage increasing in the present of co-morbidity factors (Nolan et al, 1999).

Due to these problems the ATS and CDC have suggested alternative treatment options. One such option is a daily dose of rifampicin (RMP) 4-month single-drug regimen or a daily dose of pyrazinamide (PZA)-rifampicin 4-month regimen. The RMP treatment is not recommended for HIV positive patients due to interactions with HAART treatment, but otherwise it has shown promising results for patients intolerant of INH or for those cases where INH resistance is verified or suspected. Benefits of this shorter regimen include a lower cost and also higher degrees of compliance (Jasmer et al, 2002; Menzies et al, 2004, 2008; Polesky et al, 1996; Reichman et al, 2004; Villarino et al, 1997).

Initially the PZA-RMP regimen was designed to be administered for 2 months, but due to adverse effects (serious hepatotoxicity and death) it is no longer recommended, but for some rare cases (CDC, 2001; Lecoeur, 1989; Gao, 2006) Other possible regimens that are under evaluation include a 3 month daily treatment with INH-RMP and a 3 month weekly INH-rifapentin regimen. The former has been tested in the UK and exhibits satisfactory results in terms of adverse effects and success of treatment (Ena & Valls, 2005). The latter is under study in the US, the CDC recently made public that patients on this regimen have higher compliance, satisfactory remission results compared to INH but it seems that they have increased adverse effects and also the cost of treatment is higher than the RMP regimen.

## 7. Conclusion

Latent tuberculosis is a field of great scientific interest and research possibilities. We have investigated the granuloma and its formation and 2 theories exist, a lot of the secrets still remain hidden and more evidence is needed to support either theory. In the field of diagnosis new tools are available and it remains to be seen how they will fare when tested against special populations (i.e. HIV patients which is the field of our own research as well). New guidelines for treatment are issued and those are under evaluation. Latent tuberculosis is an important public health issue, an insidious infection that can persist for years; above all, clinical suspicion is paramount for its diagnosis.

## 8. References

Ahmad S. (2010) New approaches in the diagnosis and treatment of latent tuberculosis infection *Respir Res.* Vol 11 No 1 Dec 2010 pp169

Alatas F, Alatas O, Metintas M, Ozarslan A, Erginel S & Yildirim H.(2004) Vascular endothelial growth factor levels in active pulmonary tuberculosis. *Chest.* Vol 125 No 6 Jun 2004 pp2156-9

American Thoracic Society, Centers for Disease Control and Prevention. (2000) Targeted tuberculin testing and treatment of latent tuberculosis infection. *Am J Respir Crit Care Med.* Vol 161 No 4 pt2 Apr 2000 pp221–247

Andersen P, Munk ME, Pollock JM, Doherty TM (2000) Specific immune-based diagnosis of tuberculosis. *Lancet* Vol 356 No 9235 Sep 2000 pp1099-104

Andersen P. (1997) Host responses and antigens involved in protective immunity to Mycobacterium tuberculosis. *Scand J Immunol.* Vol 45 No 2 Feb 1997 pp115-31

Arcila ML, Sánchez MD, Ortiz B, Barrera LF, García LF, Rojas M (2007) Activation of apoptosis, but not necrosis, during Mycobacterium tuberculosis infection correlated with decreased bacterial growth: role of TNF-alpha, IL-10, caspases and phospholipase A2. *Cell Immunol.* Vol 249 No 2 Oct 2007 pp80-93

Barry CE 3rd, Boshoff HI, Dartois V, Dick T, Ehrt S, Flynn J, Schnappinger D, Wilkinson RJ & Young D. (2009) The spectrum of latent tuberculosis: rethinking the biology and intervention strategies. *Nat Rev Microbiol.* Vol 7 No 12 Dec 2009 pp845-55

Beisiegel M, Mollenkopf HJ, Hahnke K, Koch M, Dietrich I, Reece ST, Kaufmann SH (2009) Combination of host susceptibility and Mycobacterium tuberculosis virulence define gene expression profile in the host *Eur J Immunol.* Vol 39 No 12 Dec 2009 pp3369-84

Bermudez LE, Goodman J (1996) Mycobacterium tuberculosis invades and replicates within type II alveolar cells *Infect Immun.* Vol 64 No 4 Apr 1996 pp1400-6

Bodnar KA, Serbina NV, Flynn JL (2001) Fate of Mycobacterium tuberculosis within murine dendritic cells. *Infect Immun.* Vol 69 No 2 Feb 2001 pp800-9

Bowdish DM, Sakamoto K, Kim MJ, Kroos M, Mukhopadhyay S, Leifer CA, Tryggvason K, Gordon S, Russell DG (2009) MARCO, TLR2, and CD14 are required for macrophage cytokine responses to mycobacterial trehalose dimycolate and Mycobacterium tuberculosis. *PLoS Pathog.*Vol 5 No 6 Jun 2009

Brodin P, Rosenkrands I, Andersen P, Cole ST & Brosch R. (2004) ESAT-6 proteins: protective antigens and virulence factors? *Trends Microbiol.* Vol 12 No11 Nov 2004 pp500-8

Cáceres N, Tapia G, Ojanguren I, Altare F, Gil O, Pinto S, Vilaplana C & Cardona PJ. (2009) Evolution of foamy macrophages in the pulmonary granulomas of experimental tuberculosis models. *Tuberculosis (Edinb).* Vol 89 No 2 Mar 2009 pp175-82

Cardona PJ. (2009) A dynamic reinfection hypothesis of latent tuberculosis infection. *Infection.* Vol 37 No 2 Apr 2009 pp80-6 Review

CDC (2001) Update: Fatal and severe liver injuries associated with rifampin and pyrazinamide for latent tuberculosis infection, and revisions in American Thoracic Society/CDC recommendations--United States, 2001. MMWR Morb Mortal Wkly Rep. Vol 50 No 34 Aug 2001 pp733-5

Center for Disease Control TB fact-sheet (n.d) http://www.cdc.gov/tb/publications/factsheets/testing/skintesting.htm

Chan J & Flynn J. The immunological aspects of latency in tuberculosis. (2004) *Clin Immunol.* Vol 110 No 1 Jan 2004 pp2-12

Cooper AM Cell-mediated immune responses in tuberculosis. *Annu Rev Immunol.* Vol 27 2009 pp393-422

Danelishvili L, Yamazaki Y, Selker J, Bermudez LE (2010) Secreted Mycobacterium tuberculosis Rv3654c and Rv3655c proteins participate in the suppression of macrophage apoptosis. *PLoS One* Vol 5 No 5 May 2010

de Jonge MI, Pehau-Arnaudet G, Fretz MM, Romain F, Bottai D, Brodin P, Honoré N, Marchal G, Jiskoot W, England P, Cole ST & Brosch R.J (2007) ESAT-6 from M. tuberculosis dissociates from its putative chaperone CFP-10 under acidic conditions and exhibits membrane-lysing activity. *Bacteriol.* Vol 189 No 16 Aug 2007 pp6028-34

Derrick SC, Morris SL (2007) The ESAT6 protein of Mycobacterium tuberculosis induces apoptosis of macrophages by activating caspase expression. *Cell Microbiol.* Vol 9 No 6 Jun 2007 pp1547-55

Diel R, Goletti D, Ferrara G, Bothamley G, Cirillo D, Kampmann B, Lange C, Losi M, Markova R, Migliori GB, Nienhaus A, Ruhwald M, Wagner D, Zellweger JP, Huitric E, Sandgren A, Manissero D (2011) Interferon-γ release assays in the diagnosis of latent M. tuberculosis infection. *Eur Respir J* Vol37 No1Jan2011 pp88-99

ECDC (2011) Guidance Use of interferon-gamma release assays in support of TB diagnosis http://ecdc.europa.eu/en/publications/Publications/1103_GUI_IGRA.pdf

ECDC (2011) Mastering the basics of TB control - Development of a handbook on TB diagnostic methods http://ecdc.europa.eu/en/publications/Publications/1105_TER_Basics_TB_control.pdf

El-Shazly S, Mustafa AS, Ahmad S & Al-Attiyah R. (2007) Utility of three mammalian cell-entry proteins of Mycobacterium tuberculosis in the serodiagnosis of tuberculosis. *Int J Tuberc Lung Dis.* Vol 11 No 6 Jun 2007 pp676–682

Ena J & Valls V (2005) Short-course therapy with rifampin plus isoniazid, compared with standard therapy with isoniazid, for latent tuberculosis infection: a meta-analysis. *Clin Infect Dis.* Vol 40 No 5 Mar 2005 pp670-6

Fuhrmann S, Streitz M & Kern F. (2008) How flow cytometry is changing the study of TB immunology and clinical diagnosis. *Cytometry A.* Vol 73 No11 Nov 2008 pp1100-6

Gao XF, Wang L, Liu GJ, Wen J, Sun X, Xie Y, Li YP (2006) Rifampicin plus pyrazinamide versus isoniazid for treating latent tuberculosis infection: a meta-analysis. Int J Tuberc Lung Dis. Vol 10 No10 Oct 2006 pp1080-90

Garton NJ, Christensen H, Minnikin DE, Adegbola RA, Barer MR (2002) Intracellular lipophilic inclusions of mycobacteria in vitro and in sputum. *Microbiology* Vol 148 No 10 Oct 2002 pp2951-8

Gehring AJ, Dobos KM, Belisle JT, Harding CV, Boom WH (2004) Mycobacterium tuberculosis LprG (Rv1411c): a novel TLR-2 ligand that inhibits human macrophage class II MHC antigen processing. *J Immunol.* Vol 15 No 173(4) Aug 2004 pp2660-8

Ghosh J, Larsson P, Singh B, Pettersson BM, Islam NM, Sarkar SN, Dasgupta S & Kirsebom LA (2009) Sporulation in mycobacteria. Proc Natl Acad Sci U S A. Vol 106 No 26 Jun 2009 pp10781-6

Gibbs JH, Ferguson J, Brown RA, Kenicer KJ, Potts RC, Coghill G, Swanson Beck J (1984) Histometric study of the localisation of lymphocyte subsets and accessory cells in human Mantoux reactions. *J Clin Pathol* Vol 37 No 11 Nov 1984 pp1227–1234

Harada K (1977) Staining mycobacteria with periodic acid-carbol-pararosanilin: principle and practice of the method. *Microsc Acta.* Vol 79 No 3 May 1977 pp224-36

Harada K, Gidoh S, Tsutsumi S (1976) Staining mycobacteria with carbolfuchsin: properties of solutions prepared with different samples of basic fuchsin. *Microsc Acta.* Vol 78 No 1 Mar 1976 pp21-27

Harboe M, Oettinger T, Wiker HG, Rosenkrands I, Andersen P (1996) Evidence for occurrence of the ESAT-6 protein in Mycobacterium tuberculosis and virulent Mycobacterium bovis and for its absence in Mycobacterium bovis BCG. *Infect Immun* Vol 64 No 1 Jan 1996 pp16-22

Harding CV, Boom WH (2010) Regulation of antigen presentation by M. tuberculosis: a role for Toll-like receptors. *Nat Rev Microbiol.* Vol 8 No 4 Apr 2010 pp296-307

Hett EC, Chao MC, Steyn AJ, Fortune SM, Deng LL & Rubin EJ (2007) A partner for the resuscitation-promoting factors of Mycobacterium tuberculosis. *Mol Microbiol.* Vol 66 No 3 Nov 2007 pp658-68

Huebner RE, Schein MF & Bass JB Jr The tuberculin skin test. *Clin Infect Dis.* Vol 17 No 6 Dec 1993 pp968-75

Ishikawa E, Ishikawa T, Morita YS, Toyonaga K, Yamada H, Takeuchi O, Kinoshita T, Akira S, Yoshikai Y, Yamasaki S (2009) Direct recognition of the mycobacterial glycolipid, trehalose dimycolate, by C-type lectin Mincle. *J Exp Med.* Vol 206 No 13 Dec 2009 pp2879-88

Jafari C, Thijsen S, Sotgiu G, Goletti D, Domínguez Benítez JA, Losi M, Eberhardt R, Kirsten D, Kalsdorf B, Bossink A, Latorre I, Migliori GB, Strassburg A, Winteroll S, Greinert U, Richeldi L, Ernst M & Lange C, Tuberculosis Network European Trialsgroup (2009) Bronchoalveolar lavage enzyme-linked immunospot for a rapid diagnosis of tuberculosis: a Tuberculosis Network European Trialsgroup study. *Am J Respir Crit Care Med.* Vol 180 No 7 Oct 2009 pp666-73

Jasmer RM, Nahid P & Hopewell PC (2002) Latent Tuberculosis Infection *N Engl J Med* Vol 347 No 23 Dec 2002 pp1860-1866

Jo EK (2008) Mycobacterial interaction with innate receptors: TLRs, C-type lectins, and NLRs. *Curr Opin Infect Dis.* Vol 21 No 3 Jun 2008 pp279-86

Jo EK, Yang CS, Choi CH, Harding CV (2007) Intracellular signalling cascades regulating innate immune responses to Mycobacteria: branching out from Toll-like receptors. *Cell Microbiol.* Vol 9 N 5 May 2007 pp1087-98

Kana BD, Gordhan BG, Downing KJ, Sung N, Vostroktunova G, Machowski EE, Tsenova L, Young M, Kaprelyants A, Kaplan G & Mizrahi V. (2008) The resuscitation-promoting factors of Mycobacterium tuberculosis are required for virulence and resuscitation from dormancy but are collectively dispensable for growth *in vitro*. *Mol Microbiol.* Vol 67 No 3 Feb 2008 pp672-84

Kenney RT, Rangdaeng S, Scollard DM (1987) Skin blister immunocytology. A new method to quantify cellular kinetics in vivo. *J Immunol Methods* Vol 97 No1 Feb 1987 pp101–110

Khader SA, Cooper AM (2008) IL-23 and IL-17 in tuberculosis. *Cytokine* Vol 41 No 2 Feb 2008 pp79–83

Kinhikar AG, Verma I, Chandra D, Singh KK, Weldingh K, Andersen P, Hsu T, Jacobs WR Jr & Laal S (2010) Potential role for ESAT6 in dissemination of M. tuberculosis via human lung epithelial cells. *Mol Microbiol.* Vol 75 No 1 Jan 2010 pp92–106

Kinhikar AG, Verma I, Chandra D, Singh KK, Weldingh K, Andersen P, Hsu T, Jacobs WR Jr, Laal S (2010) Potential role for ESAT6 in dissemination of M. tuberculosis via human lung epithelial cells. *Mol Microbiol.* Vol 75 No 1 Jan 2010 pp92-106

Kursar M, Koch M, Mittrucker HW, Nouailles G, Bonhagen K, Kamradt T, Kaufmann SH (2007) Cutting Edge: Regulatory T cells prevent efficient clearance of Mycobacterium tuberculosis. *J Immunol* Vol 178 No 5 Mar 2007 pp2661–2665

Lalor SJ, Dungan LS, Sutton CE, Basdeo SA, Fletcher JM, Mills KH (2011) Caspase-1-processed cytokines IL-1beta and IL-18 promote IL-17 production by gammadelta and CD4 T cells that mediate autoimmunity. *J Immunol. Vol* 186 No 10 May 2011 pp5738-48

Lecoeur HF, Truffot-Pernot C, Grosset JH (1989) Experimental short-course preventive therapy of tuberculosis with rifampin and pyrazinamide. *Am Rev Respir Dis.* Vol 140 No 5 Nov 1989 pp1189-93

Leyten EM, Lin MY, Franken KL, Friggen AH, Prins C, van Meijgaarden KE, Voskuil MI, Weldingh K, Andersen P, Schoolnik GK, Arend SM, Ottenhoff TH, Klein MR (2006) Human T-cell responses to 25 novel antigens encoded by genes of the dormancy regulon of Mycobacterium tuberculosis. *Microbes Infect* Vol 8 No 8 Jul 2006 pp2052–2060

Liew FY, Xu D, Brint EK & O'Neill LA (2005) Negative regulation of toll-like receptor-mediated immune responses *Nat Rev Immunol.* Vol 5 No 6 Jul 2005 pp446-58

Lin MY & Ottenhoff TH. (2008) Not to wake a sleeping giant: new insights into host-pathogen interactions identify new targets for vaccination against latent M. tuberculosis infection. *Biol Chem.* Vol 389 No 5 May 2008 pp497-511

Mahairas GG, Sabo PJ, Hickey MJ, Singh DC, Stover CK (1996) Molecular analysis of genetic differences between Mycobacterium bovis BCG and virulent M. bovis. *J Bacteriol* Vol 178 No 5 Mar 1996 pp1274-82

Master SS, Rampini SK, Davis AS, Keller C, Ehlers S, Springer B, Timmins GS, Sander P, Deretic V (2008) Mycobacterium tuberculosis prevents inflammasome activation. *Cell Host Microbe.* Vol3 No4 Apr 2008 pp224-32

Menzies D, Dion MJ, Rabinovitch B, Mannix S, Brassard P & Schwartzman K (2004) Treatment completion and costs of a randomized trial of rifampin for 4 months versus isoniazid for 9 months. *Am J Respir Crit Care Med.* Vol 170 No4 Mar 2004 pp445-9

Menzies D, Long R, Trajman A, Dion MJ, Yang J, Al Jahdali H, Memish Z, Khan K, Gardam M, Hoeppner V, Benedetti A & Schwartzman K (2008) Adverse events with 4 months of rifampin therapy or 9 months of isoniazid therapy for latent tuberculosis infection: a randomized trial. *Ann Intern Med.* Vol 149 No 10 Nov 2008 pp689-97

Menzies D, Pai M, Comstock G (2007) Meta-analysis: new tests in the diagnosis of latent tuberculosis infection: areas of uncertainty and recommendations for research. *Ann Intern Med* Vol 146 No 5 Mar 2007 pp340-54

Mishra BB, Moura-Alves P, Sonawane A, Hacohen N, Griffiths G, Moita LF, Anes E (2010) Mycobacterium tuberculosis protein ESAT-6 is a potent activator of the NLRP3/ASC inflammasome. *Cell Microbiol.* Vol 12 No 8 Aug 2010 pp1046-63

Mukamolova GV, Turapov O, Malkin J, Woltmann G & Barer MR (2010) Resuscitation-promoting factors reveal an occult population of tubercle Bacilli in Sputum. *Am J Respir Crit Care Med.* Vol 181 No 2 Jan 2010 pp174-80

Muñoz-Elias EJ, Timm J, Botha T, Chan WT, Gomez JE & McKinney JD (2005) Replication dynamics of Mycobacterium tuberculosis in chronically infected mice. *Infect Immun* Vol 73 No 1 Jan 2005 pp546–551

Neyrolles O, Hernández-Pando R, Pietri-Rouxel F, Fornes P, Tailleux L, Barris Payan JA, Pivert E, Bordat Y, Aguilar D, Prévost M-C, Petit C & Gicquel B (2006) Is adipose tissue a place for Mycobacterium tuberculosis persistence? *Pub Lib of Sci One* Vol 1 Dec 2006 pp1–9

Nigou J, Zelle-Rieser C, Gilleron M, Thurnher M, Puzo G (2001) Mannosylated lipoarabinomannans inhibit IL-12 production by human dendritic cells: evidence for a negative signal delivered through the mannose receptor. *J Immunol.* Vol 166 No 12 Jun 2001 pp7477-85.

Nolan CM, Goldberg SV & Buskin SE (1999) Hepatotoxicity associated with isoniazid preventive therapy: a 7-year survey from a public health tuberculosis clinic. *JAMA* Vol 281 No 11 Mar 1999 pp1014-8

Noss EH, Pai RK, Sellati TJ, Radolf JD, Belisle J, Golenbock DT, Boom WH, Harding CV (2001) Toll-like receptor 2-dependent inhibition of macrophage class II MHC expression and antigen processing by 19-kDa lipoprotein of Mycobacterium tuberculosis. *J Immunol.* Vol 167 No 2 Jul 2001 pp910-8.

Ohno H, Zhu G, Mohan VP, Chu D, Kohno S, Jacobs WR Jr, Chan J (2003) The effects of reactive nitrogen intermediates on gene expression in Mycobacterium tuberculosis. *Cell Microbiol.* Vol 5 No 9 Sep 2003 pp637-48.

Pai M, Zwerling A & Menzies D (2008) Systematic review: T-cell-based assays for the diagnosis of LTBI: an update. *Ann Intern Med.* Vol 149 No 3 Aug 2008 pp177-84

Pecora ND, Gehring AJ, Canaday DH, Boom WH, Harding CV (2006) Mycobacterium tuberculosis LprA is a lipoprotein agonist of TLR2 that regulates innate immunity and APC function. *J Immunol.* Vol 177 No 1 Jul 2006 pp422-9.

Peyron P, Vaubourgeix J, Poquet Y, Levillain F, Botanch C, Bardou F, Daffé M, Emile JF, Marchou B, Cardona PJ, de Chastellier C, Altare F (2008) Foamy macrophages from tuberculous patients' granulomas constitute a nutrient-rich reservoir for M. tuberculosispersistence. *PLoS Pathog.* Vol 4 No 11 Nov 2008

Pieters J (2008) Mycobacterium tuberculosis and the macrophage: maintaining a balance. *Cell Host Microbe.* Vol 3 No6 Jul 2008 pp399-407

Platt JL, Grant BW, Eddy AA, Michael AF (1983) Immune cell populations in cutaneous delayed-type hypersensitivity. *J Exp Med* Vol 158 No 4 Oct 1983 pp1227–1242.

Polesky A, Farber HW, Gottlieb DJ, Park H, Levinson S, O'Connell JJ, McInnis B, Nieves RL, Bernardo J (1996) Rifampin preventive therapy for tuberculosis in Boston's homeless. *Am J Respir Crit Care Med.* Vol 154 No 5 Nov 1996 pp1473-7

Poulter LW, Seymour GJ, Duke O, Janossy G, Panayi G (1982) Immunohistological analysis of delayed-type hypersensitivity in man. *Cell Immunol* Vol74 No2 Dec1982 pp358–369

Rees RJ & Hart PD (1961) Analysis of the host-parasite equilibrium in chronic murine TB by total and viable bacillary counts. *Br J Exp Pathol.* Vol 42 Feb 1961 pp83-8.

Reichman LB, Lardizabal A & Hayden CH (2004) Considering the role of four months of rifampin in the treatment of latent tuberculosis infection. *Am J Respir Crit Care Med.* Vol 170 No 8 Oct 2004 pp832-5

Renshaw PS, Lightbody KL, Veverka V, Muskett FW, Kelly G, Frenkiel TA, Gordon SV, Hewinson RG, Burke B, Norman J, Williamson RA & Carr MD (2005). Structure and function of the complex formed by the tuberculosis virulence factors CFP-10 and ESAT-6 *EMBO J.* Vol 24 No 14 Jul 2005 pp2491–8.

Russell DG, Cardona PJ, Kim MJ, Allain S & Altare F (2009) Foamy macrophages and the progression of the human tuberculosis granuloma. *Nat Immunol.* Vol 10 No 9 Sep 2009 pp943–948

Russell-Goldman E, Xu J, Wang X, Chan J & Tufariello JM (2008) A Mycobacterium tuberculosis Rpf double-knockout strain exhibits profound defects in reactivation from chronic tuberculosis and innate immunity phenotypes. *Infect Immun.* Vol 76 No 9 Sep 2008 pp4269-81.

Sarrazin H, Wilkinson KA & Andersson J.Rangaka MX, Radler L, van Veen K, Lange C & Wilkinson RJ (2009) Association between tuberculin skin test reactivity, the memory CD4 cell subset, and circulating FoxP3-expressing cells in HIV-infected persons. *J Infect Dis* Vol 199 No 5 Mar 2009 pp702–71

Sester M, Sotgiu G, Lange C, Giehl C, Girardi E, Migliori GB, Bossink A, Dheda K, Diel R, Dominguez J, Lipman M, Nemeth J, Ravn P, Winkler S, Huitric E, Sandgren A & Manissero D (2011) Interferon-γ release assays in the diagnosis of active TB: A systematic review and meta-analysis. *Eur Respir J* Vol 37 No 1 Jan 2011 pp100-11.

Shleeva MO, Bagramyan K, Telkov MV, Mukamolova GV, Young M, Kell DB & Kaprelyants AS (2002) Formation and resuscitation of "non-culturable" cells of Rhodococcus rhodochrous and Mycobacterium tuberculosis in prolonged stationary phase. *Microbiology* Vol 148 No 5 May 2002 pp1581–1591

TBNET Mack U, Migliori GB, Sester M, Rieder HL, Ehlers S, Goletti D, Bossink A, Magdorf K, Hölscher C, Kampmann B, Arend SM, Detjen A, Bothamley G, Zellweger JP, Milburn H, Diel R, Ravn P, Cobelens F, Cardona PJ, Kan B, Solovic J, Duarte R, Cirillo DM, & Lange C for the TBNET (2009) LTBI: latent tuberculosis infection or lasting immune responses to M. tuberculosis? A TBNET consensus statement *Eur Respir J* Vol 33 No5 May 200 pp956-973

Tufariello JM, Mi K, Xu J, Manabe YC, Kesavan AK, Drumm J, Tanaka K, Jacobs WR Jr & Chan J (2006) Deletion of the Mycobacterium tuberculosis resuscitation-promoting factor Rv1009 gene results in delayed reactivation from chronic tuberculosis. *Infect Immun.* Vol 74 No 5 May 2006 pp2985-95.

Ulrichs T, Kosmiadi GA, Trusov V, Jörg S, Pradl L, Titukhina M, Mishenko V, Gushina N & Kaufmann SH. (2004) Human tuberculous granulomas induce peripheral lymphoid follicle-like structures to orchestrate local host defence in the lung. *J Pathol.* Vol 204 No 2 Oct 2004 pp217-28.

Verhagen LM, van den Hof S, van Deutekom H, Hermans PW, Kremer K, Borgdorff MW & van Soolingen D (2011) Mycobacterial factors relevant for transmission of tuberculosis. *J Infect Dis.* Vol 203 No 9 May 2011 pp1249-55

Villarino ME, Ridzon R, Weismuller PC, Elcock M, Maxwell RM, Meador J, Smith PJ, Carson ML, Geiter LJ (1997) Rifampin preventive therapy for tuberculosis infection: experience with 157 adolescents. *Am J Respir Crit Care Med.* Vol 155 No 5 May 1997 pp1735-8

Voskuil MI, Schnappinger D, Visconti KC, Harrell MI, Dolganov GM, Sherman DR, Schoolnik GK (2003) Inhibition of respiration by nitric oxide induces a Mycobacterium tuberculosis dormancy program. *J Exp Med.* Vol 198 No 5 Sep 2003 pp 705-13.

WHO (2001) WHO warns against the use of inaccurate blood tests for active tuberculosis http://www.who.int/mediacentre/news/releases/2011/tb_20110720/en/index.html

World Health Organization Tuberculosis Fact-sheet http://www.who.int/mediacentre/factsheets/fs104/en/index.html

Zvi A, Ariel N, Fulkerson J, Sadoff JC & Shafferman A. (2008) Whole genome identification of Mycobacterium tuberculosis vaccine candidates by comprehensive data mining and bioinformatic analyses. *BMC Med Genomics.* Vol 1 May 2008 pp18

# 2

# Recent Advances in the Immunopathogenesis of *Acinetobacter baumannii* Infection

Louis de Léséleuc[1] and Wangxue Chen[1,2,*]
[1]*Institute for Biological Sciences, National Research Council Canada, Ottawa, Ontario*
[2]*Department of Biology, Brock University, St. Catharines, Ontario*
*Canada*

## 1. Introduction

Organisms belonging to the species *Acinetobacter baumannii* are capsulated coccobacillary, gram-negative bacteria. They can be found in the environment, will colonize various body tissues and food products and can persist on inanimate objects for a prolonged time period. Among the genus *Acinetobacter, A. baumannii* is the best described and most often associated with human disease and casualties. It is regarded as an opportunistic pathogen (1) and mostly targets susceptible hosts where it causes pneumonia, urinary tract infections, wound infections and meningitis. Over the last decade, we have witnessed a significant rise in the number and severity of cases of *A. baumannii* infections from hospital outbreaks as well as sporadic community-associated and wound-associated cases (2).

It is believed that the ability of *A. baumannii* to persist in the environment, notably by forming protective biofilms, as well as its remarkable spectrum of antibiotic resistance have allowed it to emerge as a particularly problematic human pathogen (3, 4). Although these attributes appear to explain the resilience of this microbe, one must remember that a large array of innocuous bacterial species, including non-pathogenic members of the *Acinetobacter* genus, can resist antibiotics and form biofilms. Hence, the question of why *A. baumannii* is such a successful and lethal pathogen becomes more pertinent. Does it display additional unique features in its interactions with the host that favour successful colonization or infection? This chapter will bring together recent research in an attempt to answer these questions. It will strive to be both informative and perhaps inspire new strategies to better control this pathogen.

## 2. Clinical manifestations of *A. baumannii* pneumonia

The major risk factor for infection with *A. baumannii*, also seen as the one that increases the overall susceptibility of the host, is the use of an invasive procedure such as mechanical

* Corresponding Author

ventilation during intensive care (5). Patients first become infected following colonization from the environment. Sources of contamination include surgical equipment, endotracheal or nasogastric tubes, catheters and previously colonized health care staff. The length of stay at the ICU has repeatedly been associated with increased risk of colonization and infection (5-7). Colonization is usually asymptomatic but will increase the likelihood of subsequent infection, which may proceed when the host natural barriers are weakened by trauma, surgery or other invasive procedures.

Respiratory tract infections constitute a major portal of entry leading to *A. baumannii* bacteremia and are almost always hospital-acquired (8). Positive blood cultures are not commonly recognized in patients with nosocomial pneumonia (8). However, pneumonia caused by this organism are significantly more frequently associated with bacteremia and result in higher mortality rates (up to 50% of cases) (8). The clinical manifestations *of A. baumannii* lung infection, both in patients and in animal models, match those of the typical bacterial pneumonia, with alveolar congestion, edema and leukocytic infiltrations. Extracellular bacteria can be readily identified and cultured from lung biopsies and post-mortem samples (8). Hence, it is alleged that bacteremia and sepsis are in most cases the final causes of death, not asphyxia and hypoxemia caused by pneumonia *per se*, although co-morbidity significantly contributes to mortality (9).

## 3. Multidrug resistance and antibiotic treatment

*Acinetobacter baumannii* has acquired resistance to many antibiotics over the last two decades (10) and the incidence of infections caused by multi-drug resistant strains of *A. baumannii* have significantly increased worldwide. This has coincided with the appearance of carbapenem-resistant *A. baumannii* strains in North America, Asia, South America, South Africa and Australia. The global dissemination of carbapenem-resistant strains of *A. baumannii* demonstrates the success of this pathogen to cause epidemic outbreaks (11). *A. baumannii* appears able to acquire antibiotic resistance through multiple mechanisms such as over-expression of bacterial efflux pumps, changes in cell wall channels (porins), acquisition of extended-spectrum β-lactamases, gene mutations and expression of certain enzymes that modify the metabolism of the antibiotic (reviewed in (12-17)). In addition, it is reported that the *A. baumannii* genome contains a "resistance island" with 45 resistance genes (18). *A. baumannii* can also rapidly acquire genetic entities for resistance, including some genes derived from other bacterial species (19). To date, *A. baumannii* strains have demonstrated resistance not only to β-lactams, aminoglycosides, fluoroquinolones, chloramphenicol, tetracycline, and rifampicin, but also to some relatively new antibiotics such as tigecycline, a novel broad-spectrum glycylcycline (20).

The emergence of multi- and pan-drug resistant *A. baumannii* strains clearly presents significant challenges to the clinical management of the infection. The antibiotic selection for those *A. baumannii* strains is very limited. Despite its potential toxicity, polymyxin B and E (colistin) are probably the most commonly used and effective antibiotics for the treatment of resistant strains of *A. baumannii* at present (12, 14-16, 21-23). Other antibiotic candidates are tigecycline and imipenem (14, 21-24) but, as discussed above, resistance to tigecycline has developed in some *A. baumannii* strains (20). To combat the multidrug resistance of *A. baumannii*, it is also a common clinical practice to prescribe several antibiotics as a combination therapy although such practice remains controversial among the medical profession (12, 24). Although antibiotic resistance and clinical treatment are the most important aspects of the management of *A. baumannii* infection, this topic is out of the main scope of this chapter. Readers are referred to some recent excellent review articles on the details of antibiotic resistance mechanisms and the advances and challenges in the development of new therapeutics for the treatment of *A. baumannii* infections (12-17, 21-23).

## 4. Experimental models of *A. baumannii* pneumonia

Many clinical cases of *A. baumannii* have been rigorously described and are very informative about the disease course, risk factors and the prevalence of antibiotic resistance and other genetic traits in the isolates. However, these studies are not experimental in nature and are based on retrospective analysis of hospital-based cases. Thus, they generally fail to establish a causal relationship between the attributes of a given isolate and disease transmissibility, severity and clinical course, which define virulence. Knowledge of virulence factors can help both identify potentially dangerous pathogens before they strike and help develop new methods of control or treatments. Unfortunately, to date, aside from antibiotic-resistance genes, few virulence factors have been identified in *A. baumannii* (Table 1), despite wide variation in the ability of different laboratory strains and clinical isolates to cause disease in experimental models (25, 26). In addition, although a number of host factors have been examined for their potential involvement in the control of *A. baumannii*, only a few have been shown to play a role in resistance to infection (Table 2).

| Contributing factors | Model | Route of infection | Readout | Reference |
|---|---|---|---|---|
| LPS | Serum sensitivity | *in vitro* | Resistance to normal human serum | (38) |
| LPS | Rat soft tissue<br>Human serum | Subcutaneous<br>*in vitro* | Bacterial growth/survival | (39) |
| Many genes and loci including urease | *Caenorhabditis elegans*<br>*Dictyostelium discoideum* | *in vitro* | Killing, egg count<br>Plaque assay | (34) |
| *OmpA* | A549 epithelial cells | *in vitro* | Adherence, apoptosis | (42) |
| *OmpA* | A549 epithelial cells<br>Mouse | *in vitro*<br>Intratracheal | Invasion<br>Blood counts | (43) |
| PBP-7/8 | Rat soft tissue<br>Rat pneumonia<br>Human serum | Subcutaneous<br>Intratracheal<br>*in vitro* | Bacterial growth/survival | (46) |
| Phospholipase D | Human serum<br>Epithelial cells<br>Mouse | *in vitro*<br>*in vitro*<br>Intranasal | Growth<br>Invasion<br>Blood counts | (47) |
| *pmrB* | Mouse | Intraperitoneal | Survival, microbial growth in spleen | (35) |
| *ptk, epsA*, capsule | Human ascites fluid<br>Rat soft tissue | *in vitro*<br>Subcutaneous | Bacterial growth/survival | (40) |
| *RecA* | Macrophages<br>Mouse | *in vitro*<br>Intraperitoneal | Bacterial survival<br>Mortality | (50) |

Table 1. Identified virulence factors of *A. baumannii*

| Resistance factors | Model | Route of infection | Readout | Noncontributing factors | Reference |
|---|---|---|---|---|---|
| Acute-phase response and serum amyloid A (negative effect) | Mouse, turpentine acute phase model | Intranasal | Lung bacterial burdens | TNF-α | (69) |
| CD14, TLR4 | Mouse | Intranasal | Bacterial growth | TLR2 | (65) |
| Complement | Human serum | *in vitro* | Bacterial growth/survival | N/A | (29, 45) |
| NADPH oxidase | Mouse | Intranasal | Lung and spleen bacterial burdens | NOS2 | (71) |
| Neutrophils | Mouse, systemic | Intraperitoneal | Survival, bacterial burden in organs | Sex, strain, IL-17A, KC | (25) |
| Neutrophils, MIP-2 | Mouse, two strains | Intranasal | Lung and spleen bacterial burdens | N/A | (28, 70) |

Table 2. Identified host factors that are important in resistance to *A. baumannii* infection

The most widely used model for the study of *A. baumannii* virulence and host responses is based on the mouse (26-28). It has been exploited to study pneumonia as well as septicaemia caused by *A. baumannii* and was successful in identifying or validating both microbial virulence and host resistance factors. Overall, conventional mice (such as C57BL/6 and BALB/c) show relatively high resistance to respiratory infection with *A. baumannii*. Mice inoculated intranasally with up to $10^8$ viable *A. baumannii* develop an acute, self-limiting bronchopneumonia and infected mice generally clear the infection by 96 hours after inoculation (28). Moreover, the infection is usually limited to the respiratory tract with minimal systemic dissemination. As expected, treatment of mice with immunosuppressive drugs (such as cyclophosphamide) greatly exacerbate the infection and can convert an otherwise self-limiting infection into a lethal one (27). In addition, a rat model has been established and used to study both pneumonia and soft tissue injury (29). Human studies are so far limited to bactericidal assays using serum or ascites fluid and the use of human peripheral blood mononuclear cells and various epithelial cell lines (29-33). More basic *in vivo* models involving inhibition of *Caenorhabditis elegans* and *Dictyostelium discoideum* were employed for screening the virulence of multiple *A. baumannii* transposon insertional mutants (34). In many studies, more than one aspect of virulence was explored to generate a more complete picture.

## 5. Virulence factors of *A. baumannii*

One of the defining attributes of *A. baumannii*, both biologically and clinically, is its ability to resist a number of antibiotic classes. It is often debated whether antibiotic resistance genes can be considered virulence factors. On the one hand, they do contribute to the capacity of the pathogen to cause disease by resisting treatment. On the other hand, they do not directly affect the natural course of the infection and only play a role when an exogenous chemotherapeutic compound is administered. However, this distinction is blurred when that resistance to antibiotics impacts on virulence in the absence of the antibiotic. For instance it was reported that colistin-resistant *A. baumannii* isolates show a general lower fitness as assessed by animal mortality and bacterial burdens in organs (35). The mutation conferring antibiotic resistance was mapped to the *pmrB* gene. The *pmrABC* operon mediates resistance to colistin and other polymyxins through modification of the lipid A portion of LPS (36). Polymyxins bind to LPS; resistance can occur by the complete loss of lipid A through disruption of the biosynthetic genes, yielding LPS-deficient, Gram-negative bacteria (37). LPS was identified in at least two independent studies as contributing to bacterial virulence. It was first found to be important for serum resistance whereas capsular polysaccharide was dispensable (38). This was recently reproduced and further investigated in a wound infection model where LPS was found to be important for bacterial growth and survival (39). Hence, it is not surprising that downregulation of LPS as a means to resist polymyxins will significantly impact the virulence of the organism and might explain the low prevalence of colistin resistance in clinical isolates (21).

While capsular polysaccharides may not be required for serum resistance, the capsule was shown to be a major contributor to virulence since the growth of capsule-deficient variants of *A. baumannii* was attenuated in human ascites fluid and in a wound infection model (40). Hence, it is evident that different virulence factors may be manifest at distinct stages and physiological locations of the infection. Another iteration of that concept is found with outer membrane protein A (AbOmpA), a porin-like protein of *A. baumannii* which appears to mediate multiple functions. This protein is homologous to OmpA proteins from *Enterobacteria* and outer membrane protein F (OprF) of *Pseudomonas sp.* (41). AbOmpA was reported to mediate cytotoxicity in human HEp-2 cells (32) and dendritic cells (33). It also mediates interaction and invasion of lung epithelial cells as wells as biofilm formation on abiotic surfaces (42, 43). Whether these *in vitro* events (attachment, invasion and apoptosis) are important for *in vivo* virulence is still uncertain. Moreover, AbOmpA was recently shown to play a role in iron metabolism, another feature that may impact virulence (44). In this regard, blood dissemination of OmpA-deficient bacteria was less pronounced in the mouse pneumonia model (43), suggesting that this protein influences virulence at one or many of the steps leading to bacteremia. One of these steps could be resistance to complement-mediated lysis (45).

Random transposon mutagenesis has the potential to provide a large amount of unbiased information about microbial virulence. In the last few years, this approach has been adapted for the study of *A. baumannii* physiology and pathogenesis. The first study reported by Michael G. Smith and colleagues (2007) combined high-density pyrosequencing with transposon mutagenesis and identified a number of putative pathogenicity loci (34). Their screen was based on inhibition of *Dictyostelium* and *Caenorhabditis elegans* by *A. baumannii* mutants. They reported that a large proportion of the pathogen's genome consisted of foreign DNA and found six islands associated with virulence. This underlined once more the ability of this pathogen to adapt and evolve by acquiring genetic material for antibiotic resistance and virulence. While informative, this screen was only a first step since the mutants were not complemented nor were they tested in a mammalian model. More recently, Russo *et al.* (2009) identified a putative low-molecular-mass penicillin-binding protein 7/8 (PBP-7/8) as a virulence gene based on serum sensitivity and validated it in the rat models of pneumonia and soft tissue infection (46). PBP-7/8 affects cell morphology and is suspected to play a role in peptidoglycan synthesis and cell wall structure. A similar mutagenesis study using serum sensitivity as the readout and pneumonia as the validation step identified phospholipase D (PLD) as a *bona fide* virulence factor (47). Interestingly, PLD is also associated with virulence in *Neisseria gonorrhoeae* (48) and *Corynebacterium pseudotuberculosis* (49). Hence this enzyme could be used as a drug target for the design of novel antimicrobials.

Another bacterial enzyme that was recently shown to play a role in virulence is recA (50). This protein was found not only to mediate DNA repair in *A. baumannii* but also played a role in desiccation resistance, prevented killing inside macrophages as well as contributed to mouse lethality. It may be argued that such a pleotropic protein may not qualify as an authentic virulence factor, for which the defining function is to ensure development inside a live host independently of *in vitro* or environmental fitness. Nevertheless, recA shows promise as a specific antimicrobial target and its implication in virulence underscores the importance of a microorganism's DNA repair pathway in the battle between host and pathogen.

## 6. Biofilm formation

One of the hallmark features of the *Acinetobacter* genus is the ability to form biofilms on animate and inanimate surfaces. Biofilm formation is associated with bacterial persistence in chronic diseases and in the environment; however, it is not yet clear whether production of biofilms by *A. baumannii* is involved in virulence. A high level of heterogeneity has been observed between isolates with respect to biofilm formation, which could not be correlated with virulence or disease severity (51-53). Moreover, biofilm production and adherence to airway epithelial cells is also observed at similar frequencies in low virulence species of Acinetobacters (30). Nevertheless, biofilm formation may contribute to disease transmissibility by promoting survival of *A. baumannii* on surgical instruments, catheters and external body surfaces and enabling colonization. It is likely that a combination of features, including the various virulence factors, resistance to multiple antibiotics and general hospital infection management etc., make *A. baumannii* a successful clinical pathogen.

## 7. Iron acquisition

One last feature that is under scrutiny is the role of iron in *A. baumannii* pathogenesis. Iron is a redox metal essential to most life forms; it is a component of many enzymes and factors such as ribonucelotide reductase (54) and the cytochromes of the aerobic electron transport chain (55). Although abundant inside the body, iron is usually found in association with host macromolecules like heme and transferrin and, thus, is not readily available to bacteria. As a result, *A. baumannii* must develop strategies to capture and retain iron for its survival and growth. Using a proteomics-based approach, 58 proteins were found to be differentially expressed in *A. baumannii* in response to iron modulation, including AbOmpA (44). Although the importance of iron acquisition in pathogenesis has not been experimentally established, this suggests that *A. baumannii* has evolved sophisticated regulatory mechanisms to respond to iron deprivation which are meant to ensure survival in the host, where this metal is scarce.

The production of siderophores is one strategy used by the pathogen to grow under iron-limiting conditions (56, 57). Siderophores are small secreted molecules that bind iron with high affinity and can be taken up by bacteria as a way to scavenge trace iron from their surroundings. The siderophore produced by the *A. baumannii* type strain 19606 was termed "acinetobactin" (58). It is structurally related to the siderophore produced by *Vibrio anguillarum* and resembles catechol-type siderophores such as the enterobactins (59). Of note, *A. baumannii* isolates often differ in the structure of the siderophores and other iron acquisition factors they express (60). Another way that *A. baumannii* can acquire iron in the circulation is by utilizing hemin, a salt of heme generated from the breakdown of hemoglobin (61). Conversely, *A. baumannii* cannot use hemoglobin itself (61) and does not bind the iron transporter transferrin (57), unlike other gram-negative bacteria such as *Neisseria* and *Moraxella* (62).

The importance of iron metabolism was also supported by the discovery that a novel monobactam-class antibiotic, BAL30072, is particularly active against *A. baumannii* when tested against a panel of pathogenic gram-negative species (63, 64). BAL30072 is a catecholic β-lactam that binds iron and acts as a siderophore (63). Under iron-restricted conditions such as those encountered *in vivo,* the molecule would be taken up efficiently by the bacteria's siderophore capture machinery, acting as a Trojan horse to deliver the antibiotic inside the cell. Hence it is possible that a microorganism with a high avidity for iron and siderophores, such as *A. baumannii,* might be more easily targeted and killed by antibiotics of this class. As a bonus, resistance might appear by downregulating siderophore uptake but only at the expense of *in vivo* fitness.

## 8. Host resistance factors

Like *A. baumannii* virulence factors, host factors important for protection against *A. baumannii* infection are still largely unexplored. It is generally recognized that immunocompromised individuals are much more likely to become infected by *A. baumannii,* an opportunistic pathogen by most definitions (1). As such, the host innate immune system is generally successful in controlling the pathogen and that only when it fails does the infection progress, such as upon barrier disruption, severe stress or immunosuppressive drug treatment. Identification of host immune cells and molecules that are critical for resistance could help us better deal with these deadly infections by monitoring those factors and boosting or supplementing them as the need arises.

Infections with *A. baumannii* are characterised by an acute, rapid progression. The host appears to either control the infection or becomes overwhelmed by it. This implies that innate immunity plays a major role in the control of this pathogen. Indeed, CD14 and TLR4, members of the innate immune system and the LPS sensing pathway, have been shown to be essential for resistance to *A. baumannii* infection in a knockout mouse model, while TLR2 appeared to counteract the robustness of the induced innate immunity (65).

The importance of LPS sensing would be consistent with a strong, protective pro-inflammatory reaction against the pathogen. Paradoxically, trauma and postsurgical patients mounting a strong systemic acute-phase response are more susceptible to *A. baumannii* infections (66-68). Experimentally, an acute-phase response elicited in mice with turpentine or by direct injection of exogenous serum amyloid A protein reduced pulmonary inflammation and neutrophil migration during *A. baumannii* pneumonia (69). This treatment ultimately led to enhanced susceptibility in the mice. This phenomenon might explain part of the immunosuppression that permits the microbe to successfully infect hospital patients. Hence, control of *A. baumannii* probably requires a targeted and self-limiting inflammatory response.

Major effectors of the innate inflammatory response, neutrophils play a critical role in the control of *A. baumannii* infection, as would be expected when dealing with extracellular bacteria. They are rapidly recruited to the lungs after infection and contribute to its resolution. Early animal models of *A. baumannii* pneumonia used cyclophosphamide to render mice neutropenic (24, 27) which might have increased the magnitude of bacterial replication *in vivo*, although this was not addressed directly. The role of neutrophils was not formally investigated until much later when it was found that antibody-mediated depletion of neutrophils resulted in an acute lethal infection in mice that was associated with enhanced bacterial burdens in the lung and extrapulmonary dissemination to the spleen (28). Conversely, enhanced pulmonary recruitment of neutrophils by intranasal supplementation of the chemoattractant MIP-2 promoted clearance of the pathogen (28).

The importance of neutrophils and of the regulation of their trafficking was reinforced when it was shown that A/J mice are more susceptible to *A. baumannii* compared to C57BL/6 mice due to a delayed and weaker neutrophil recruitment (70). Strain differences in host responses are common and may lead to genetic studies uncovering novel resistance factors. However, the choice of strains, route of infection and measurements might be of prime importance since another study did not report differences between their experimental mouse strains when doing Intraperitoneal injections (25) while a third found differences in mortality but not in lung bacteriology when comparing three murine strains (27).

The role of neutrophils was further investigated at the molecular level to determine what effector functions were required for clearance of *A. baumannii*. It was found that NADPH phagocyte oxidase expressed in neutrophils played a major role in extrapulmonary dissemination of *A. baumannii* whereas the contribution of inducible nitric oxide synthase (NOS2) was minor (71). This is consistent with evidence that NOS2 may be predominantly restricted to the control of intracellular pathogens (72). Other factors suspected to play a role such as sex, IL-17A and the chemokine KC (CXCL1) were also ruled out (25). Still unresolved is the role of the lung macrophages and epithelial cells in the initial recognition of the pathogen and subsequent recruitment of neutrophils. Are these cell types and others involved in recruiting neutrophils to the site of infection? Is infection of epithelial cells essential for the translocation of the pathogen into the circulation? Many of the initial steps of *A. baumannii* infection remain unexplored.

In the bloodstream, *A. baumannii* would encounter other hurdles to infection and dissemination. Blood contains a number of innate immune components that can restrict bacterial growth and even kill a large proportion of infecting microorganisms. Human serum is bactericidal or bacteriostatic to most strains of *A. baumannii* and this was shown to be mediated by complement (29, 45). The alternative complement pathway is responsible for killing the bacteria (45, 51). Interestingly, serum resistance in some strains was explained by the binding of Factor H, an inhibitor of this pathway, to *A. baumannii* outer membrane proteins, including AbOmpA (45). However, this is not a universal phenomenon since binding to Factor H was not observed in another set of serum-resistant isolates (51).

There is clearly a substantial amount of variability in both the serum sensitivity of the pathogen and the bactericidal activity of sera from different individuals (38, 73). This could be due to past exposures and the presence of circulating antibodies. Lifelong exposure to *Acinetobacter* species from the environment might confer some low level of immunity to the pathogen. Indeed, both active and passive immunization using an inactivated whole cell vaccine are very effective at preventing *A. baumannii* infection in mice (74). This could explain why blood from naïve mice does not show any inhibitory activity towards *A. baumannii* (unpublished observations) and would suggest that blood does not contain significant natural defences against the pathogen, a state that could prove detrimental to the susceptible, naïve host.

## 9. Conclusion

*Acinetobacter baumannii* presents an array of features that make it a particularly troublesome pathogen. Similar to other emerging gram-negative bacilli like *Pseudomonas aeruginosa* and *Klebsiella pneumonia*, its quick rise in the past decades is probably the result of an ability to rapidly evolve and acquire new genetic material for virulence and antibiotic resistance. The multidrug resistance of several isolates of *A. baumannii* can be traced back to multiple events including downregulation of porins, expression of drug-inactivating enzymes and target alterations (75). Furthermore, the ability of *A. baumannii* to form biofilms allows it to persist on abiotic surfaces, a first step in disease transmission. When it finds an appropriate niche, such as the lung, it rapidly multiplies and creates a localized infection or colonization. If this infection is not contained effectively because of treatment failure or ineffective host defense mechanism, bacteremia will rapidly progress which may prove fatal.

Fast-growing in nature and able to overwhelm host defences, *A. baumannii* has a limited but effective set of virulence factors. One of them, AbOmpA, appears to simultaneously mediate host cell invasion, serum resistance and iron uptake, three potential prerequisites to virulence. This protein could therefore be a prime candidate for therapies targeting virulence mechanisms. Phospholipase D and recA are other candidates with an even wider spectrum that could benefit treatments of other infections. Other strategies targeting iron acquisition by the microbe could also prove successful. On the host side, boosting the activity of innate immunity such as neutrophils, or at least maintaining their proper numbers and function, could help slow or halt the progress of the pathogen.

Given the wide variation in the clinical success, biofilm formation, disease pathogenesis and antibiotic resistance profiles of *A. baumannii* isolates, it is currently difficult to pinpoint which steps and factors are really essential for virulence and which merely modulate it. More research needs to be conducted to better understand pathogenesis, preferably in experimentally controlled conditions involving characterised hosts and bacteria. Given enough information, the ultimate goal would be to predict the course and outcome of the disease when encountering an unknown isolate, in order to take appropriate measures. Another benefit would be to identify new therapeutic targets to supplement and perhaps replace the shrinking arsenal of chemotherapeutic agents at our disposal.

## 10. Acknowledgements

We wish to thank our current and past laboratory members and collaborators for their contributions in *Acinetobacter* research project and thank Ms. Rhonda KuoLee for her assistance in the preparation of this manuscript.

## 11. References

[1] Bergogne-Berezin E, Towner KJ. Acinetobacter spp. as nosocomial pathogens: microbiological, clinical, and epidemiological features. Clin Microbiol Rev. 1996 Apr;9(2):148-65.

[2] Van Looveren M, Goossens H. Antimicrobial resistance of Acinetobacter spp. in Europe. Clin Microbiol Infect. 2004 Aug;10(8):684-704.

[3] Go ES, Urban C, Burns J, Kreiswirth B, Eisner W, Mariano N, et al. Clinical and molecular epidemiology of acinetobacter infections sensitive only to polymyxin B and sulbactam. Lancet. 1994 Nov 12;344(8933):1329-32.

[4] Villers D, Espaze E, Coste-Burel M, Giauffret F, Ninin E, Nicolas F, et al. Nosocomial Acinetobacter baumannii infections: microbiological and clinical epidemiology. Ann Intern Med. 1998 Aug 1;129(3):182-9.

[5] Baran G, Erbay A, Bodur H, Onguru P, Akinci E, Balaban N, et al. Risk factors for nosocomial imipenem-resistant Acinetobacter baumannii infections. Int J Infect Dis. 2008 Jan;12(1):16-21.

[6] Jamulitrat S, Thongpiyapoom S, Suwalak N. An outbreak of imipenem-resistant Acinetobacter baumannii at Songklanagarind Hospital: the risk factors and patient prognosis. J Med Assoc Thai. 2007 Oct;90(10):2181-91.

[7] Lee SO, Kim NJ, Choi SH, Hyong Kim T, Chung JW, Woo JH, et al. Risk factors for acquisition of imipenem-resistant Acinetobacter baumannii: a case-control study. Antimicrob Agents Chemother. 2004 Jan;48(1):224-8.

[8] Magret M, Lisboa T, Martin-Loeches I, Manez R, Nauwynck M, Wrigge H, et al. Bacteremia is an independent risk factor for mortality in nosocomial pneumonia: a prospective and observational multicenter study. Crit Care. 2011 Feb 16;15(1):R62.

[9] Cisneros JM, Rodriguez-Bano J. Nosocomial bacteremia due to Acinetobacter baumannii: epidemiology, clinical features and treatment. Clin Microbiol Infect. 2002 Nov;8(11):687-93.

[10] Fournier PE, Richet H. The epidemiology and control of Acinetobacter baumannii in health care facilities. Clin Infect Dis. 2006 Mar 1;42(5):692-9.

[11] Higgins PG, Dammhayn C, Hackel M, Seifert H. Global spread of carbapenem-resistant Acinetobacter baumannii. J Antimicrob Chemother. 2010 Feb;65(2):233-8.

[12] Munoz-Price LS, Weinstein RA. Acinetobacter Infection. N Engl J Med. 2008 March 20, 2008;358(12):1271-81.

[13] Towner KJ. Acinetobacter: an old friend, but a new enemy. J Hosp Infect. 2009 Dec;73(4):355-63.

[14] Maragakis LisaÂ L, Perl TrishÂ M. Antimicrobial Resistance: Acinetobacter baumannii: Epidemiology, Antimicrobial Resistance, and Treatment Options. Clinical Infectious Diseases. 2008;46(8):1254-63.

[15] Gootz TD, Marra A. Acinetobacter baumannii: an emerging multidrug-resistant threat. Expert review of anti-infective therapy. 2008 Jun;6(3):309-25.

[16] Dijkshoorn L, Nemec A, Seifert H. An increasing threat in hospitals: multidrug-resistant Acinetobacter baumannii. Nature reviews. 2007 Dec;5(12):939-51.

[17] Gaynes R, Edwards JR. Overview of nosocomial infections caused by gram-negative bacilli. Clin Infect Dis. 2005 Sep 15;41(6):848-54.

[18] Fournier PE, Vallenet D, Barbe V, Audic S, Ogata H, Poirel L, et al. Comparative genomics of multidrug resistance in Acinetobacter baumannii. PLoS Genet. 2006 Jan;2(1):e7.

[19] Ribera A, Ruiz J, Vila J. Presence of the Tet M determinant in a clinical isolate of Acinetobacter baumannii. Antimicrob Agents Chemother. 2003 Jul;47(7):2310-2.

[20] Navon-Venezia S, Leavitt A, Carmeli Y. High tigecycline resistance in multidrug-resistant Acinetobacter baumannii. J Antimicrob Chemother. 2007 Apr;59(4):772-4.
[21] Livermore DM, Hill RL, Thomson H, Charlett A, Turton JF, Pike R, et al. Antimicrobial treatment and clinical outcome for infections with carbapenem- and multiply-resistant Acinetobacter baumannii around London. Int J Antimicrob Agents. 2009 Jan;35(1):19-24.
[22] Michalopoulos A, Falagas ME. Treatment of Acinetobacter infections. Expert Opin Pharmacother. 2010 Apr;11(5):779-88.
[23] Murray CK, Hospenthal DR. Treatment of multidrug resistant Acinetobacter. Current opinion in infectious diseases. 2005 Dec;18(6):502-6.
[24] Wolff M, Joly-Guillou ML, Farinotti R, Carbon C. In vivo efficacies of combinations of beta-lactams, beta-lactamase inhibitors, and rifampin against Acinetobacter baumannii in a mouse pneumonia model. Antimicrob Agents Chemother. 1999 Jun;43(6):1406-11.
[25] Breslow JM, Meissler JJ, Jr., Hartzell RR, Spence PB, Truant A, Gaughan J, et al. Innate Immune Responses to Systemic Acinetobacter baumannii infection in Mice: Neutrophils, but not IL-17, Mediate Host Resistance. Infect Immun. 2011 May 16.
[26] Eveillard M, Soltner C, Kempf M, Saint-Andre JP, Lemarie C, Randrianarivelo C, et al. The virulence variability of different Acinetobacter baumannii strains in experimental pneumonia. J Infect. 2010 Feb;60(2):154-61.
[27] Joly-Guillou ML, Wolff M, Pocidalo JJ, Walker F, Carbon C. Use of a new mouse model of Acinetobacter baumannii pneumonia to evaluate the postantibiotic effect of imipenem. Antimicrob Agents Chemother. 1997 Feb;41(2):345-51.
[28] van Faassen H, KuoLee R, Harris G, Zhao X, Conlan JW, Chen W. Neutrophils play an important role in host resistance to respiratory infection with Acinetobacter baumannii in mice. Infect Immun. 2007 Dec;75(12):5597-608.
[29] Russo TA, Beanan JM, Olson R, MacDonald U, Luke NR, Gill SR, et al. Rat pneumonia and soft-tissue infection models for the study of Acinetobacter baumannii biology. Infect Immun. 2008 Aug;76(8):3577-86.
[30] de Breij A, Dijkshoorn L, Lagendijk E, van der Meer J, Koster A, Bloemberg G, et al. Do biofilm formation and interactions with human cells explain the clinical success of Acinetobacter baumannii? PLoS One. 2010;5(5):e10732.
[31] March C, Regueiro V, Llobet E, Moranta D, Morey P, Garmendia J, et al. Dissection of host cell signal transduction during Acinetobacter baumannii-triggered inflammatory response. PLoS One. 2010;5(4):e10033.
[32] Choi CH, Lee EY, Lee YC, Park TI, Kim HJ, Hyun SH, et al. Outer membrane protein 38 of Acinetobacter baumannii localizes to the mitochondria and induces apoptosis of epithelial cells. Cell Microbiol. 2005 Aug;7(8):1127-38.
[33] Lee JS, Choi CH, Kim JW, Lee JC. Acinetobacter baumannii outer membrane protein A induces dendritic cell death through mitochondrial targeting. J Microbiol. 2010 Jun;48(3):387-92.
[34] Smith MG, Gianoulis TA, Pukatzki S, Mekalanos JJ, Ornston LN, Gerstein M, et al. New insights into Acinetobacter baumannii pathogenesis revealed by high-density pyrosequencing and transposon mutagenesis. Genes Dev. 2007 Mar 1;21(5):601-14.

[35] Lopez-Rojas R, Dominguez-Herrera J, McConnell MJ, Docobo-Perez F, Smani Y, Fernandez-Reyes M, et al. Impaired virulence and in vivo fitness of colistin-resistant Acinetobacter baumannii. J Infect Dis. 2011 Feb 15;203(4):545-8.

[36] Arroyo LA, Herrera CM, Fernandez L, Hankins JV, Trent MS, Hancock RE. The pmrCAB operon mediates polymyxin resistance in Acinetobacter baumannii ATCC 17978 and clinical isolates through phosphoethanolamine modification of Lipid A. Antimicrob Agents Chemother. 2011 Jun 6.

[37] Moffatt JH, Harper M, Harrison P, Hale JD, Vinogradov E, Seemann T, et al. Colistin resistance in Acinetobacter baumannii is mediated by complete loss of lipopolysaccharide production. Antimicrob Agents Chemother. 2010 Decv;54(12):4971-7.

[38] Garcia A, Solar H, Gonzalez C, Zemelman R. Effect of EDTA on the resistance of clinical isolates of Acinetobacter baumannii to the bactericidal activity of normal human serum. J Med Microbiol. 2000 Nov;49(11):1047-50.

[39] Luke NR, Sauberan SL, Russo TA, Beanan JM, Olson R, Loehfelm TW, et al. Identification and characterization of a glycosyltransferase involved in Acinetobacter baumannii lipopolysaccharide core biosynthesis. Infect Immun. 2010 May;78(5):2017-23.

[40] Russo TA, Luke NR, Beanan JM, Olson R, Sauberan SL, MacDonald U, et al. The K1 capsular polysaccharide of Acinetobacter baumannii strain 307-0294 is a major virulence factor. Infect Immun. 2010 Sep;78(9):3993-4000.

[41] Gribun A, Nitzan Y, Pechatnikov I, Hershkovits G, Katcoff DJ. Molecular and structural characterization of the HMP-AB gene encoding a pore-forming protein from a clinical isolate of Acinetobacter baumannii. Curr Microbiol. 2003 Nov;47(5):434-43.

[42] Gaddy JA, Tomaras AP, Actis LA. The Acinetobacter baumannii 19606 OmpA protein plays a role in biofilm formation on abiotic surfaces and in the interaction of this pathogen with eukaryotic cells. Infect Immun. 2009 Aug;77(8):3150-60.

[43] Choi CH, Lee JS, Lee YC, Park TI, Lee JC. Acinetobacter baumannii invades epithelial cells and outer membrane protein A mediates interactions with epithelial cells. BMC Microbiol. 2008;8:216.

[44] Nwugo CC, Gaddy JA, Zimbler DL, Actis LA. Deciphering the iron response in Acinetobacter baumannii: A proteomics approach. J Proteomics. 2010 Jan 1;74(1):44-58.

[45] Kim SW, Choi CH, Moon DC, Jin JS, Lee JH, Shin JH, et al. Serum resistance of Acinetobacter baumannii through the binding of factor H to outer membrane proteins. FEMS Microbiol Lett. 2009 Dec;301(2):224-31.

[46] Russo TA, MacDonald U, Beanan JM, Olson R, MacDonald IJ, Sauberan SL, et al. Penicillin-binding protein 7/8 contributes to the survival of Acinetobacter baumannii in vitro and in vivo. J Infect Dis. 2009 Feb 15;199(4):513-21.

[47] Jacobs AC, Hood I, Boyd KL, Olson PD, Morrison JM, Carson S, et al. Inactivation of phospholipase D diminishes Acinetobacter baumannii pathogenesis. Infect Immun. 2010 May;78(5):1952-62.

[48] Edwards JL, Apicella MA. Neisseria gonorrhoeae PLD directly interacts with Akt kinase upon infection of primary, human, cervical epithelial cells. Cell Microbiol. 2006 Aug;8(8):1253-71.

[49] McNamara PJ, Bradley GA, Songer JG. Targeted mutagenesis of the phospholipase D gene results in decreased virulence of Corynebacterium pseudotuberculosis. Mol Microbiol. 1994 Jun;12(6):921-30.
[50] Aranda J, Bardina C, Beceiro A, Rumbo S, Cabral MP, Barbe J, et al. The Acinetobacter baumannii RecA protein in the repair of DNA damage, antimicrobial resistance, general stress response, and virulence. J Bacteriol. 2011 Jun 3.
[51] King LB, Swiatlo E, Swiatlo A, McDaniel LS. Serum resistance and biofilm formation in clinical isolates of Acinetobacter baumannii. FEMS Immunol Med Microbiol. 2009 Apr;55(3):414-21.
[52] Cevahir N, Demir M, Kaleli I, Gurbuz M, Tikvesli S. Evaluation of biofilm production, gelatinase activity, and mannose-resistant hemagglutination in Acinetobacter baumannii strains. J Microbiol Immunol Infect. 2008 Dec;41(6):513-8.
[53] Wroblewska MM, Sawicka-Grzelak A, Marchel H, Luczak M, Sivan A. Biofilm production by clinical strains of Acinetobacter baumannii isolated from patients hospitalized in two tertiary care hospitals. FEMS Immunol Med Microbiol. 2008 Jun;53(1):140-4.
[54] Brown NC, Eliasson R, Reichard P, Thelander L. Nonheme iron as a cofactor in ribonucleotide reductase from E. coli. Biochem Biophys Res Commun. 1968 Mar 12;30(5):522-7.
[55] Rainnie DJ, Bragg PD. The effect of iron deficiency on respiration and energy-coupling in Escherichia coli. J Gen Microbiol. 1973 Aug;77(2):339-49.
[56] Echenique JR, Arienti H, Tolmasky ME, Read RR, Staneloni RJ, Crosa JH, et al. Characterization of a high-affinity iron transport system in Acinetobacter baumannii. J Bacteriol. 1992 Dec;174(23):7670-9.
[57] Actis LA, Tolmasky ME, Crosa LM, Crosa JH. Effect of iron-limiting conditions on growth of clinical isolates of Acinetobacter baumannii. J Clin Microbiol. 1993 Oct;31(10):2812-5.
[58] Yamamoto S, Okujo N, Sakakibara Y. Isolation and structure elucidation of acinetobactin, a novel siderophore from Acinetobacter baumannii. Arch Microbiol. 1994;162(4):249-54.
[59] Dorsey CW, Tomaras AP, Connerly PL, Tolmasky ME, Crosa JH, Actis LA. The siderophore-mediated iron acquisition systems of Acinetobacter baumannii ATCC 19606 and Vibrio anguillarum 775 are structurally and functionally related. Microbiology. 2004 Nov;150(Pt 11):3657-67.
[60] Dorsey CW, Beglin MS, Actis LA. Detection and analysis of iron uptake components expressed by Acinetobacter baumannii clinical isolates. J Clin Microbiol. 2003 Sep;41(9):4188-93.
[61] Zimbler DL, Penwell WF, Gaddy JA, Menke SM, Tomaras AP, Connerly PL, et al. Iron acquisition functions expressed by the human pathogen Acinetobacter baumannii. Biometals. 2009 Feb;22(1):23-32.
[62] Beddek AJ, Schryvers AB. The lactoferrin receptor complex in Gram negative bacteria. Biometals. 2010 Jun;23(3):377-86.
[63] Mushtaq S, Warner M, Livermore D. Activity of the siderophore monobactam BAL30072 against multiresistant non-fermenters. J Antimicrob Chemother. 2010 Feb;65(2):266-70.

[64] Page MG, Dantier C, Desarbre E. In vitro properties of BAL30072, a novel siderophore sulfactam with activity against multiresistant gram-negative bacilli. Antimicrob Agents Chemother. 2010 Jun;54(6):2291-302.
[65] Knapp S, Wieland CW, Florquin S, Pantophlet R, Dijkshoorn L, Tshimbalanga N, et al. Differential roles of CD14 and toll-like receptors 4 and 2 in murine Acinetobacter pneumonia. Am J Respir Crit Care Med. 2006 Jan 1;173(1):122-9.
[66] Ayan M, Durmaz R, Aktas E, Durmaz B. Bacteriological, clinical and epidemiological characteristics of hospital-acquired Acinetobacter baumannii infection in a teaching hospital. J Hosp Infect. 2003 May;54(1):39-45.
[67] Keen EF, 3rd, Robinson BJ, Hospenthal DR, Aldous WK, Wolf SE, Chung KK, et al. Incidence and bacteriology of burn infections at a military burn center. Burns. 2010 Jun;36(4):461-8.
[68] Caricato A, Montini L, Bello G, Michetti V, Maviglia R, Bocci MG, et al. Risk factors and outcome of Acinetobacter baumanii infection in severe trauma patients. Intensive Care Med. 2009 Nov;35(11):1964-9.
[69] Renckens R, Roelofs JJ, Knapp S, de Vos AF, Florquin S, van der Poll T. The acute-phase response and serum amyloid A inhibit the inflammatory response to Acinetobacter baumannii Pneumonia. J Infect Dis. 2006 Jan 15;193(2):187-95.
[70] Qiu H, KuoLee R, Harris G, Chen W. High susceptibility to respiratory Acinetobacter baumannii infection in A/J mice is associated with a delay in early pulmonary recruitment of neutrophils. Microbes Infect. 2009 Oct;11(12):946-55.
[71] Qiu H, Kuolee R, Harris G, Chen W. Role of NADPH phagocyte oxidase in host defense against acute respiratory Acinetobacter baumannii infection in mice. Infect Immun. 2009 Mar;77(3):1015-21.
[72] Chakravortty D, Hensel M. Inducible nitric oxide synthase and control of intracellular bacterial pathogens. Microbes Infect. 2003 Jun;5(7):621-7.
[73] Liao CH, Sheng WH, Chen YC, Hung CC, Wang JT, Chang SC. Predictive value of the serum bactericidal test for mortality in patients infected with multidrug-resistant Acinetobacter baumannii. J Infect. 2007 Aug;55(2):149-57.
[74] McConnell MJ, Pachon J. Active and passive immunization against Acinetobacter baumannii using an inactivated whole cell vaccine. Vaccine. 2010 Dec 10;29(1):1-5.
[75] Gootz TD. The global problem of antibiotic resistance. Crit Rev Immunol. 2010;30(1):79-93.

# 3

# Pulmonary Nontuberculous Mycobacterial Infections in the State of Para, an Endemic Region for Tuberculosis in North of Brazil

Ana Roberta Fusco da Costa[1,2], Maria Luiza Lopes[1],
Maísa Silva de Sousa[2], Philip Noel Suffys[3],
Lucia Helena Messias Sales[4] and Karla Valéria Batista Lima[1]
[1]*Evandro Chagas Institute, Bacteriology Section*
[2]*Federal University of Para, Tropical Medicine Nucleus*
[3]*Oswaldo Cruz Institute, Oswaldo Cruz Foundation*
[4]*Federal University of Para, Department of Integrative Medicine*
*Brazil*

## 1. Introduction

Traditionally, *Mycobacterium* species are divided in those belonging to the *Mycobacterium tuberculosis* complex (MTBC), *M. leprae* and the nontuberculous or atypical mycobacteria (NTM), the latter consisting of either rapid (RGM) or slow growing (SGM) species, forming colonies, respectively, within seven days of culture or requiring longer incubation time (Runyon, 1959). Among the RGM are the *M. chelonae* complex, including *M. chelonae, M. abscessus, M. mucogenicum, M. salmoniphilum, M. bolletii* and *M. massiliense* (Brown-Elliot & Wallace, 2002; Whipps et al., 2007) and the *M. fortuitum* complex, including *M. fortuitum, M. peregrinum, M. septicum, M. mageritense, M. houstonense* and *M. boenikei* (Adékambi & Drancourt, 2004), containing the NTM commonly encountered in human specimens. Clinically important SGM are the *M. avium* complex (MAC), which include *M. avium, M. intracellulare, M. colombiense* and *M. chimaera* (Tortoli, 2003; Tortoli et al., 2004).

Until now, 130 *Mycobacterium* species, with a considerable variability in pathogenicity have been described, being isolated from natural water reservoirs and drinking water distribution systems in buildings, hospitals, household plumbing, hot tubs, spas, building aerosols, boreal forest soils and peats, acidic, brown-waters swamps, potting soils and metal removal fluid systems (Tortoli, 2009; Euzéby, 2011, Falkinham, 2009). The lack of evidence for person-to-person transmission suggests that the environment is the most likely source of NTM infection (Marra & Daley, 2002).

Unlike the bacterial species that belong to the MTBC, NTM are commonly present in the environment and when isolated from human specimens, may either be (i) contaminants during preparation of sputum cultures in the laboratory, (ii) colonizing organisms of the airways without causing disease or (iii) infectious organisms and causing disease and it is not always easy to distinguish between these situations (Griffith et al., 2007). In the case of real infection with NTM, clinical syndromes are either lymphadenitis, pulmonary or cutaneous infection or disseminated disease, chronic pulmonary infection being the most common (Katoch, 2004; Piersimoni & Scarparo, 2009; Tortoli, 2009). Such NMT infections are frequently observed in immune-compromised patients in developed nations but also in immune-competent individuals with pre-existing structural pulmonary diseases (Griffith et al., 2007; Jeong et al., 2004; Jarzembowski & Young, 2008; Bodle et al., 2008; Glassroth, 2008; Sexton & Harrison, 2008; Griffith, 2010).

The diagnosis of NTM pulmonary disease is often difficult due to the overwhelming presence of environmental organisms, to the indolent nature of disease and the diversity of, mostly, nonspecific clinical symptoms. Therefore, guidelines and criteria for diagnosis of NTM pulmonary disease have been published (American Thoracic Society, 1997; British Thoracic Society, 2000) followed by the publication of a recent update of more lenient criteria (Griffith et al., 2007). Even so, these recommendations do not seem to be satisfactory as most patients with pulmonary disease due to NTM do not match these criteria (Marras et al., 2007; van Ingen et al., 2009). Also, in endemic countries for tuberculosis (TB), the pulmonary disease form is caused also by infection with organisms of the MTBC, presenting similar clinical symptoms. In addition, diagnostic procedures for pulmonary TB are sputum smear microscopy for acid-fast bacilli (AFB) and X-ray, not differentiating between *Mycobacterium* to the species level. Nonetheless, several case reports and studies on the prevalence of pulmonary disease caused by NTM in North America, Europe and Japan have been published during the last years (Good, 1980; Tsukamura et al., 1988; von Reyn et al., 1993; Falkinham, 2002; Kobashi & Matsushima, 2007; Iseman & Marras, 2008; Billinger et al., 2009; Thomson, 2010; Kendall et al., 2011).

The impact, magnitude and regional dimension of NTM infections in countries where TB is endemic is hardly known (Gopinath & Singh, 2010), such as the case in Brazil, where most cases of infectious NTM have been reported in the southeastern region and, more specifically, in São Paulo (Barreto & Campos, 2000; Ueki et al., 2005; Zamarioli et al., 2008; Pedro et al., 2008). In the Amazon region, North of Brazil, little epidemiological information on this matter is available (da Costa et al., 2009).

We therefore studied the frequency and diversity of NTM isolates, obtained from pulmonary specimens from residents of the Pará State, during a twelve year period.

## 2. Material and methods

### 2.1 Study setting and patients

All *Mycobacterium* isolates evaluated were obtained from sputum samples (n = 119) and bronchial washings (n = 9) from individuals with clinical symptoms of pulmonary TB and residents of the State of Pará, North Brazil (Fig. 1). The study included samples of patients from whom NTM was isolated from at least once, and this between January 1999 and December 2010, at the Evandro Chagas Institute, a reference center for the diagnosis of infections with *Mycobacterium*. Patient records were reviewed to assess the frequency of isolation and clinical relevance of the presence of NTM and the diagnosis for NTM lung infection was based on the diagnostic criteria published by the American Thoracic Society (Griffith et al., 2007) (Table 1).

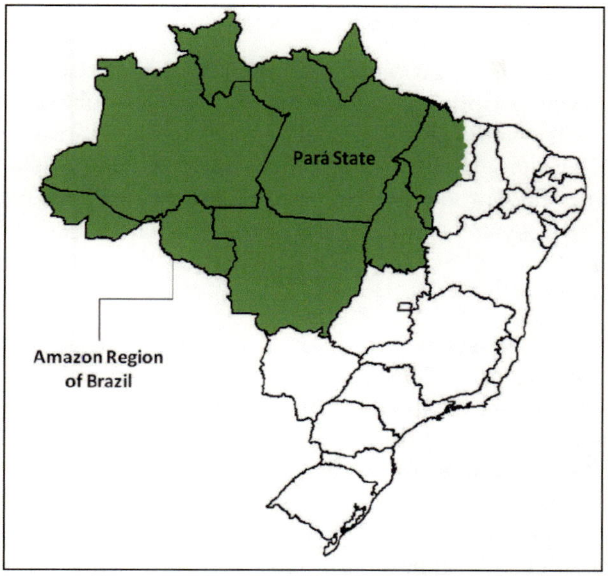


Fig. 1. Geographic localization of the Pará State, Amazon Region of Brazil.

| |
|---|
| **Clinical and radiographic analysis** |
| - Pulmonary symptoms that include nodular or cavitary opacities on chest radiograph; multifocal bronchiectasis with multiple small nodules on a high resolution computed tomography (HRCT) scan; lack of abnormalities suggestive for other disease. |
| **Microbiologic analysis** |
| - Positive culture from at least two separate expectorated sputum samples, when initial sputum samples are AFB negative, consider repeated sputum AFB smears and cultures or positive culture results from at least one bronchial wash or lavage |
| **Histopathologic analysis** |
| - Transbronchial or other lung biopsy with mycobacterial histopathologic features (granulomatous inflammation or AFB) and positive culture for NTM. |

Table 1. American Thoracic Society diagnostic criteria on NTM pulmonary disease (Griffith ei al., 2007).

### 2.2 *Mycobacterium* cultures and isolates

Pulmonary specimens were decontaminated using the N-acetyl-L-cysteine-sodium hydroxide procedure (Webb, 1962; Brasil, 2008), inoculated into Lowenstein-Jensen (LJ) medium (Difco, France) and incubated at 35 to 37°C in the absence of light for at least six weeks or until colonies appeared. Conventional procedures for distinguishing between organisms of the MTBC and of the NTM group included macroscopic analysis of aspect of colonies, which MTBC have a rough aspect resemble breadcrumbs or cauliflowers, detection of cord factor from MTBC by Ziehl-Neelsen stain, and the growth inhibition test in medium containing 0.5 mg/mL para-nitrobenzoic acid, a specific inhibitor of MTBC, all according to Kubica (1973).

### 2.3 Sequence analysis and phylogenetic analysis

Sequencing of part of the 16S ribosomal RNA (16S rRNA) and 65-kilodalton heat shock protein (*hsp65*) genes was performed as described by previous publications (Kim et al., 2005; Shin et al., 2006). After verification of PCR products on agarose gel Seakem LE 1% (Cambrex, United Kingdom), these were purified using the SNAP TM gel purification kit (Invitrogen). The amplified products were direct sequenced by using both forward and reverse primers of each system and the BigDye Terminator v3.1 cycle sequencing kits (Applied Biosystems, Foster City, CA) and analyzed on an ABI3130 sequencer (Applied Biosystems, Tokyo, Japan).

The 16S rRNA and *hsp65* sequences were aligned using the multiple-alignment algorithm of the Bioedit software (version 7.0.9; Tom Hall [http://www.mbio.ncsu.edu/BioEdit/bioedit.html]) with the closest relatives retrieved from the GenBank database across of the Basic Local Alignment Search Tool (BLAST, URL: http://www.ncbi.nlm.nih.gov/ BLAST/) and the Ribosomal Differentiation of Medical Microorganisms RIDOM database (RIDOM, URL: http://rdna.ridom.de/). Phylogenetic trees were constructed from the presently-defined 16S rRNA or *hsp65* sequences separately using the neighbor-joining algorithm, including sequences of a selection of NTM-type strains, retrieved from GenBank (accession numbers in parenthesis next to the species names in Figs.3 and 4). For this, we used the Kimura's 2-parameter distance correction model and MEGA software (Version 4.0; Tamura et al. [http://www.megasoftware.net/]). Bootstrap analysis (1,000 repeats) was applied using the *Tsukamurela paurometabola* (KCTC 9821) sequences as an out-group. The GenBank accession numbers for the *Mycobacterium* sequences determined in this study included the following: FJ590454-FJ590472, HM056080- HM056113 for the 16S rRNA, and FJ536235- FJ536253, HM056114- HM056147 for the *hsp65* gene.

### 2.4 Statistical analysis

Statistical data were derived by using the nonparametric chi-square test and the Fisher exact test, where appropriate. P values less than 0.05 was considered significant. Statistical analysis was performed with the BioEstat software (version 5.0; Ayres et al. [http: www.mamiraua.org.br]).

## 3. Results

### 3.1 Patients and NTM isolates

Between 1999 and 2010, *Mycobacterium* isolates were recovered from respiratory specimens of 1,580 patients, that were suspected of having pulmonary TB. Among these, 92% (1,453 cases) were infected with MTBC; from the rest (8%, 128 patients) we obtained 249 NTM isolates. Among the NTM-positive patients studied, 57.5% (n=73) presented at least two positive sputum cultures for the same species, or presented at least one bronchial wash positive culture and suffered therefore from infections as defined by the criteria of ATS (Griffith et al., 2007). The clinical significance of NTM pulmonary isolation among 1999-2010 is shown in Fig.2.

The remaining 55 patients could not be confirmed to suffer from NMT infection because (i) only a single sputum sample was collected and delivered to the laboratory (47 patients); (ii)

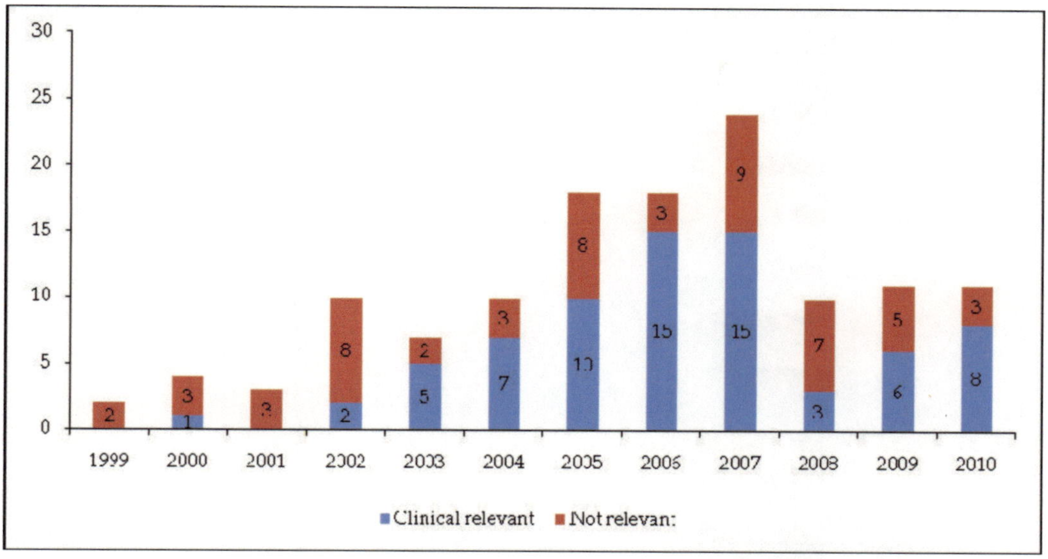


Fig. 2. Frequency of NTM isolation from clinical pulmonary specimens of patients from Pará State, Brazil, 1999-2010.

one sample was culture-positive and the others were culture-negative (five cases) or (iii) NTM were found in some patients who were also TB-positive (three patients). Distribution of species according clinical relevance and years of isolation is show in Tab.2 and Fig.3.

| Species | Clinical relevant | | Not relevant | | Total | |
|---|---|---|---|---|---|---|
| | Patients | Isolates | Patients | Isolates | Patients | Isolates |
| *M. massiliense* | 20 | 39 | 8 | 8 | 28 | 47 |
| *M. simiae complex* | 14 | 44 | 5 | 5 | 19 | 49 |
| *M. intracellulare* | 11 | 32 | 6 | 6 | 17 | 38 |
| *M. avium* | 10 | 28 | 12 | 12 | 22 | 40 |
| *M. bolletii* | 4 | 14 | 0 | 0 | 4 | 14 |
| *M. abscessus* | 3 | 8 | 1 | 1 | 4 | 9 |
| *M. colombiense* | 3 | 9 | 2 | 2 | 5 | 11 |
| *M. kansasii* | 2 | 3 | 0 | 0 | 2 | 3 |
| *M. simiae* | 2 | 4 | 1 | 1 | 3 | 5 |
| *M. fortuitum* | 1 | 6 | 18 | 18 | 19 | 24 |
| *M. scrofulaceum* | 1 | 3 | 0 | 0 | 1 | 3 |
| *M. szulgai* | 1 | 2 | 0 | 0 | 1 | 2 |
| *M. terrae* | 1 | 2 | 0 | 0 | 1 | 2 |
| *M. parascrofulaceum* | 0 | 0 | 1 | 1 | 1 | 1 |
| *M. smegmatis* | 0 | 0 | 1 | 1 | 1 | 1 |
| Total | 73 | 194 | 55 | 55 | 128 | 249 |

Table 2. Clinical significance of NTM isolated in Pará State, Brazil, 1999-2010.

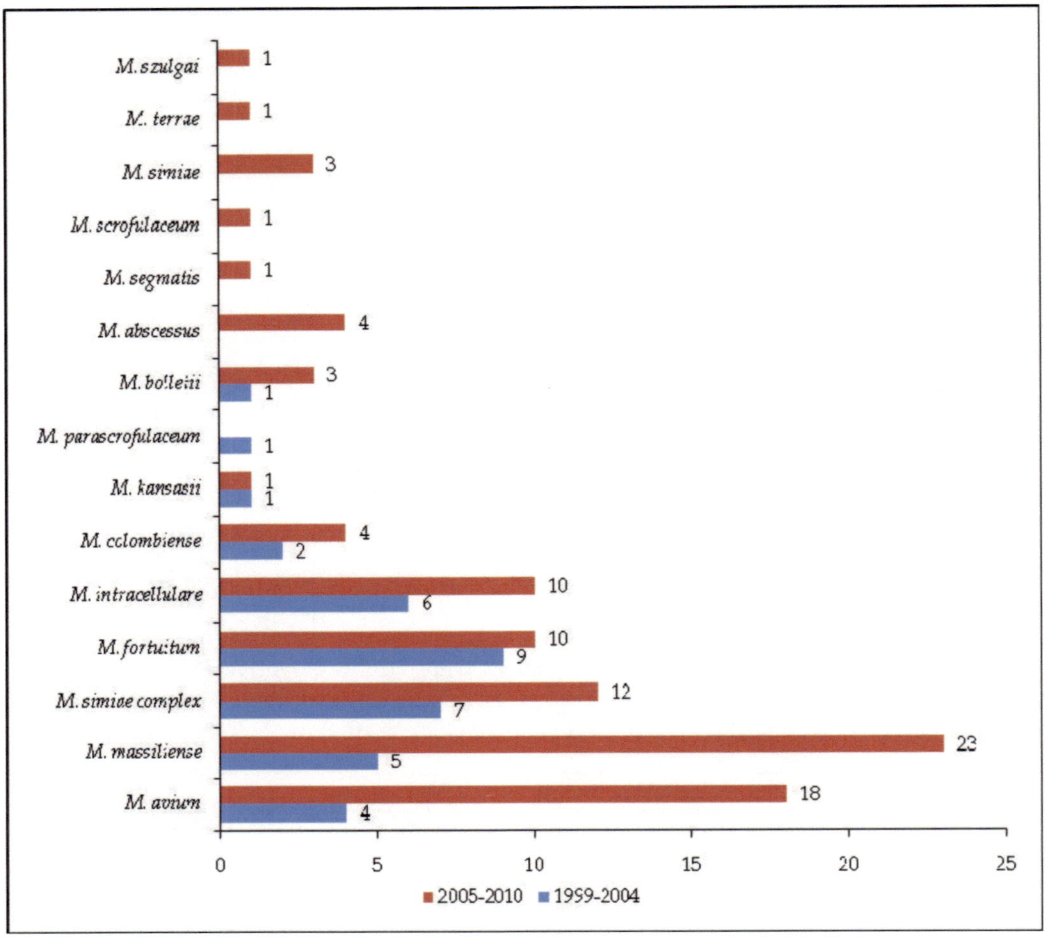


Fig. 3. Frequency of isolation of nontuberculous *Mycobacterium* species between the 1999-2003 and 2004-2010 periods in Pará State, Brazil.

Among the 73 patients with bacteriological ATS criteria for NMT infection, 64.4% (n=47; $p$ = 0,03) were females and more detailed analysis of their treatment history revealed that 72 had previously been unsuccessfully treated for TB, using the first-line multidrug therapy scheme; one patient had been diagnosed as suffering from allergic bronchitis and therefore submitted to corticosteroid therapy. After confirmation of NTM infection, 70 patients were submitted to a daily regimen of clarithromycin (500-1,000 mg) and ethambutol (25 mg/kg) for 12 months. No therapy information was available for the patient infected with *M. fortuitum* and for the two cases with *M. kansasii*. Treatment outcome was not available for all cases but patients infected with members of the *M. simiae* complex did not present clinical improvement and at the end of our study period, one had died due to progression of disease.

All of the patients described above presented respiratory complaints consistent with TB while additional symptoms were observed (Table 3). Bronchiectasis sequelae occasionally associated with hemoptysis in patients infected with *M. abscessus* ($n$=1), *M. bolletii* ($n$=2), *M.*

| Species | Gender | | Clinical characteristics | Total |
|---|---|---|---|---|
| | Male | Female | | |
| *M. massiliense* | 6 | 14 | chronic cough (20); sputum (20); chest pain (20); hemoptysis (5); dyspnea; loss weight (3) | 20 |
| *M. simiae* complex | 4 | 10 | chronic cough (14); sputum (14); chest pain (14) weight loss (14); fever (3); hemoptysis (10); malaise (14); dyspnea (3); down syndrome (1); fatigue (2) | 14 |
| *M. intracellulare* | 5 | 6 | chronic cough (11); sputum (11); chest pain (3) | 11 |
| *M. avium* | 2 | 8 | chronic cough (10); sputum (10); chest pain (10); HIV (1); gastroesophageal reflux disease (1) | 10 |
| *M. bolletii* | 3 | 1 | chronic cough (4); hemoptysis (2); decreased lung volume (1); fever (1); loss weight (1) | 4 |
| *M. abscessus* | 1 | 2 | chronic cough (3); sputum (3); hemoptysis (1); dyspnea (1); corticosteroid-immunosuppressed (1) | 3 |
| *M. colombiense* | 2 | 1 | chronic cough (3); chest pain (3) | 3 |
| *M. kansasii* | 1 | 1 | chronic cough (2); chest pain (2) | 2 |
| *M. simiae* | 0 | 2 | chronic cough (2); chest pain (2) | 2 |
| *M. fortuitum* | 1 | 0 | chronic cough (1); chest pain (1) | 1 |
| *M. scrofulaceum* | 0 | 1 | chronic cough (1); chest pain (1) | 1 |
| *M. szulgai* | 0 | 1 | chronic cough (1); chest pain (1) | 1 |
| *M. terrae* | 1 | 0 | chronic cough (1); chest pain (1) | 1 |

Table 3. Clinical characteristics of patients with NTM pulmonary infection from Pará State, Brazil, 1999-2010.

*massiliense* (*n*=5) and *M. simiae* complex (*n*=10) while chronic cough was observed among patients, independent of the infecting *Mycobacterium* species. The interval between the onset of signs and symptoms and a definitive diagnosis of NTM infection was greater than 12 months, being more pronounced in cases with *M. simiae* complex isolates, reporting the presence of symptoms for at least 24 months.

### 3.2 NTM Identification on the genetic level

Based on 16S rRNA gene analysis, the majority of the NTM species isolated from patients could be grouped into three clades, containing sequences from either *M. avium*, *M. chelonae* or *M. simiae* complexes (Fig. 4).

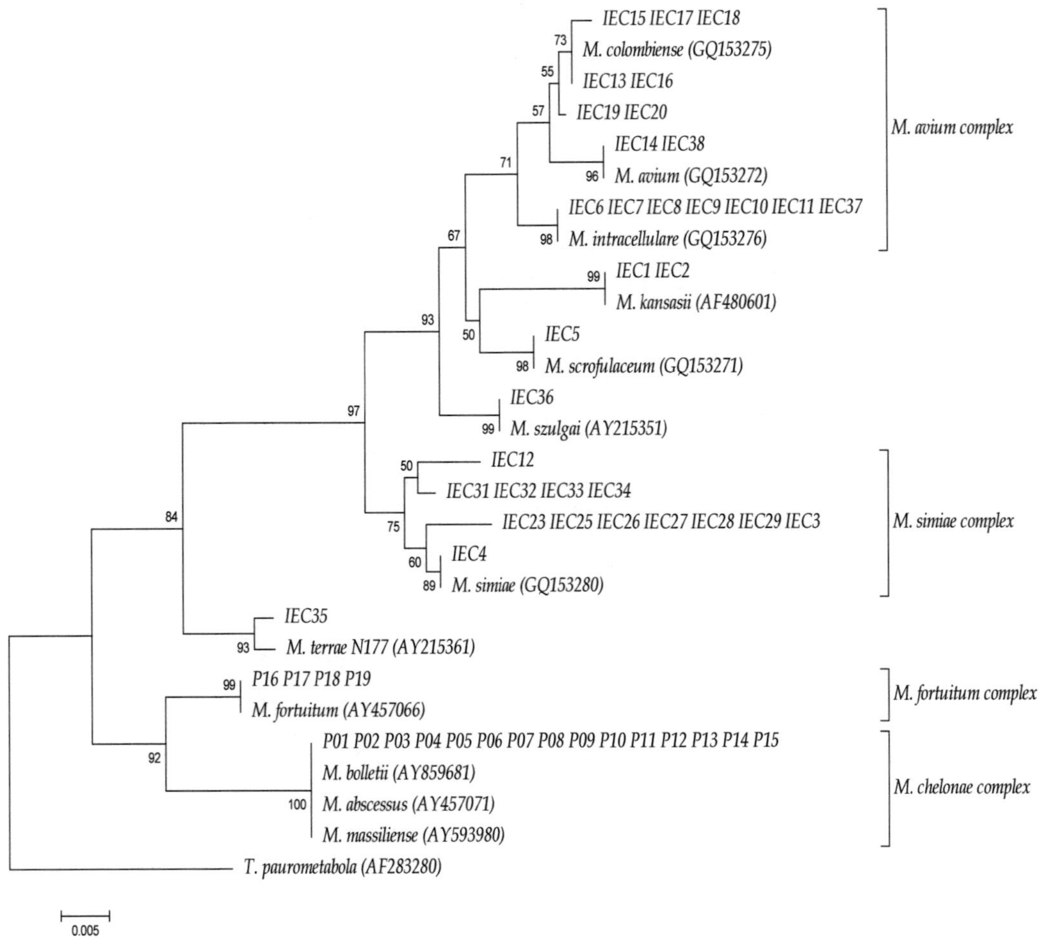


Fig. 4. Relationships between sequences from the type strains and the NTM isolated presently, inferred from partial 16S rRNA gene. Phylogenetic tree was constructed by neighbor-joining method and Kimura's 2-parameter distance correction model. The support of each branch, as determined from 1000 bootstrap samples, is indicated by the value at each node (as a percentage). *T. paurometabola* KCTC 9821 was used as outgroup.

Upon sequence analysis of part of the *hsp65* gene, we observed a higher genetic diversity than that of the 16S rRNA gene; nonetheless, the phylogenetic tree based on *hsp65* gene sequence analysis had the same global topology as that based on 16S rRNA gene (Fig. 5).

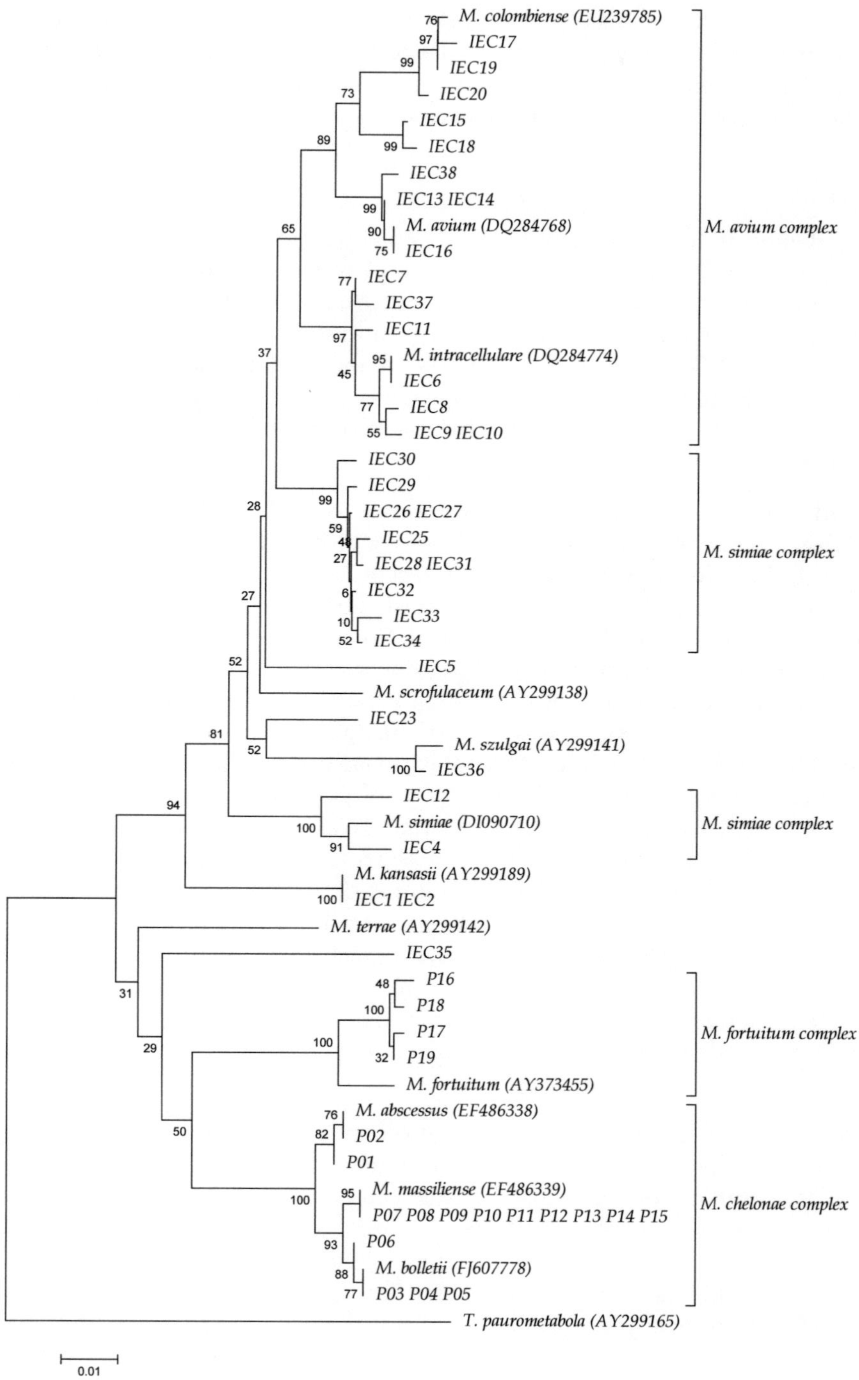


Fig. 5. Relationships between sequences from the type strains and the NMT isolated presentlty, as inferred from partial *hsp65* sequences. Phylogenetic tree was constructed as described above.

Among the 249 infectious isolates, 200 NMT sequences, derived from 108 patients, had already been described elsewhere and characteristic for 14 NMT species, the other 49 sequences derived from 19 cases were unpublished in public databases and all phylogenetically classified into the *M. simiae* complex.

## 4. Discussion

This study demonstrates that among 1,453 cases that were diagnosed between 1999 and 2010 as suffering from pulmonary TB, presence of NTM was observed in 128 (8%) of these and infection with such species proven to cause disease in 73 cases (5%). It was observed a steady increase in the number of NTM isolates during the study period, which was more pronounced from 2004 on, when an increase in the demand of culture for AFB at the Evandro Chagas Institute was the case. This latter could be due either to the increase of the physicians' sensitivity to occurrence of NTM infections in this region and/or to an increase of infection with NMT of the population.

In this study, significantly more females were infected with NTM, and this is contrary to most published data, presenting males as the major risk group for pulmonary NMT disease (Marras & Daley, 2002). However, some recent reports also demonstrated a female predominance (Freeman et al., 2007; Cassid et al., 2009; Prevot et al., 2010; Wintrop et al., 2010), in concordance with the recent data of Chan & Iseman (2010), describe a higher immune susceptibility of women to NTM pulmonary disease. In addition, when stratifying to the NMT species level, it was observed that gender associated infection was even more pronounced in the case of *M. massiliense* (70% females), *M. simiae* complex (71%) and *M. avium* (66%). Griffith et al. (2003) found a predominance of females (65%) among 154 cases of pulmonary disease by RGM, while descriptions of particular forms of pulmonary disease caused by MAC in women have been reported (Wallace, 1994; Reich & Johnson, 1995). Further studies are needed to elucidate the reasons for female susceptibility. Roughly 40% (*n*=55) of the patients with NTM-positive cultures did not meet the diagnostic criteria for NTM pulmonary infection but this does not necessarily mean that the presence of NMT is not the cause of disease. Unfortunately, due to lack of follow-up of patients, it cannot confirm this presently. There is little known about the pathophysiology of NTM-related lung disease what makes it difficult to be certain that colonization is not an indolent or even a slowly-progressive infection. Therefore, such cases need to remain under observation and seek expert consultation (Griffith et al., 2007).

Among the cases with confirmation of NMT infection as a cause of disease, mostly, previous diagnosis and treatment of TB was observed, none demonstrating improvement following treatment. Misdiagnosis of NTM infections as caused by members of the MTBC leads to unsuccessful treatment with anti-TB drugs and because clinicians experiment with various TB therapies without considering a culture-based test, there is a considerable delay in detection of NTM. This is even more a matter of concern in high prevalence countries of TB such as Brazil, where mostly, symptomatic patients with sputum smear positive for acid-fast bacilli are treated with anti-TB drugs without being testing for NTM-related disease, except when co-infected with HIV (Brasil, 2005).

In Brazil, it was common until 2009, to start second line treatment without performing culture test for NTM, when no improvement during the first round of TB treatment was observed. The high level of pulmonary NTM that was misdiagnosed as TB strongly suggests the need for a different strategy of TB control in the state of Para.

In most countries, NTM-related disease, unlike TB, do not need to be reported unless they are healthcare-associated infections. Therefore, information on the frequency and diversity of NTM infections are usually obtained from laboratory records and surveillance studies (Marras et al., 2007; Parrish et al., 2008). To determine the true epidemiological status of NTM pulmonary disease, well designed population-based studies are needed. However, the financial burden on public health care system in developing countries makes it difficult to perform such surveillance studies. Therefore, laboratory procedures such as the introduction of both liquid and solid culture systems and use of molecular methods such as PCR restriction analysis (PRA) in reference laboratories could be an alternative for more knowledge and improvement of diagnose accuracy in those regions.

Sequence analysis has contributed to the recent description of several new *Mycobacterium* species and more precise identification and taxonomy of members of this genus. Genotypic taxonomy is typically based on the detection of highly conserved regions within the genome that harbor hypervariable sequences in which species-specific deletions, insertions, or replacements of single nucleotides are present in 16S rRNA, *hsp65* gene and more recently on a fragment of the gene coding for the beta sub-unit of RNA polymerase (*rpoB*) are also contributing to this field, mostly for RGM (da Costa et al., 2009; da Costa et al, 2010). Several amplification molecular methods, have been proposed to correct NTM identification, including specific DNA probes (AccuProbe: GenProbe, Inc., San Diego, CA, U.S.A) and PRA method based on 16S rRNA (Domenech et al., 1994), 16S-23S rRNA internal transcribed spacer (ITS) (Roth et al., 1998), *hsp65* (Telenti et al., 1993), *rpoB* (Lee et al., 2000), cold-shock protein gene (*dnaJ*) (Takewaki et al., 1994), DNA repair protein gene (*recA*) (Blackwood et al., 2000) and elongation factor Tu gene (*tuf*) (Shin et al., 2009), but all have limitations as the variety of mycobacteria to be identified (da Costa et al., 2010a, b).

Based on the 16S rRNA and *hsp65* nucleotide sequences, we observed that the most frequent NTM isolates from our pulmonary samples were those of the *M. avium*, *M. chelonae* and *M. simiae* complexes. The most common NTM were *M. massiliense*, *M. intracellulare*, followed by *Mycobacterium* sp. from *M. simiae* complex. When compared with reports on NMT infections observed in other studies reported on Brazilian NTM cases, the species diversity and frequency is quite particular to the Para State, suggesting that environmental characteristics as temperature, pH and substrate composition may influence the geographical distribution of species. Our findings are in concordance with the fact that isolates of the *M. simiae* complex are rarely observed in other regions of Brazil.

There are few publications describing NTM in the Amazon region or Brazil. Barreto and Campos (2000) found 35 patients with NTM and showed that isolates of the *M. avium* complex, *M. terrae* and *M. fortuitum* were most common in samples collected between 1994 and 1999 in North of Brazil. A study that evaluated respiratory samples of non-indigenous and indigenous patients from Amazonas State with suspected pulmonary TB identified 19 patients with NTM infection, but the study did not report the identity of the isolates at the species level (Santos et al., 2006). A recent study by da Costa et al. (2009), showed that the *M. chelonae* complex, which includes the *M. massiliense* species, is the most frequent cause of pulmonary infections by RGM in Pará State, Amazon region of Brazil, similar to our observations. Unlikely, in Brazilian southeast, *M. kansasii* and *M. avium* represented the most frequent type of NTM associated with pulmonary infections between 1991 and 1997 in the state of São Paulo (Ueki et al., 2005; Zamarioli et al. 2008; Pedro et al., 2008).

In contrast to other parts of the world, the species variability found in the present study is different. In countries from Latin America like Colombia, MAC, *M. chelonae* and *M. fortuitum* were the NTM isolated with more frequency (León, 1998), while MAC was most frequently isolated from argentinian HIV patients (Di Lonardo, 1995). MAC and *M. kansasii* were predominant in North America, some countries of Europe and South Africa (Griffith et al., 2007). In Asia, MAC, *M. abscessus* and *M. chelonae* were frequently isolated from pulmonary samples (Simons et al., 2011). The knowledge on diversity and epidemiology of species NTM associated to pulmonary in specific region is important because either: (i) it allows the adequate choice of laboratory methods for diagnosis (ii) it allows to recognize the species associated to disease; and (iii) it supplies information that will serve to improve the organization of health service net to attend these patients.

Perhaps the most important finding of this study was the identification of *M. simiae* complex members as the predominant cause of pulmonary infections. In fact, roughly 20% ($n$=16) of the pulmonary infections were caused by members of the *M. simiae* complex and among these, 14 belonged to an unidentified taxon (n=14). Currently, this taxonomic group is made up of 17 species including *M. simiae, M. genavense, M. intermedium, M. interjectum, M. lentiflavum, M. triplex, M. heidelbergense, M. kubicae, M. palustre, M. montefiorense, M. florentinum, M. sherrisii, M. parmense, M. parascrofulaceum, M. saskatchewanense, M. stomatepiae* and *M. europaeum* (Tortoli, 2003, 2006; Tortoli et al., 2010). However, among these species, only *M. simiae* is recognized as a real cause of pulmonary infections, as reported in areas such as the Southwest of the United States, Israel and Cuba (Griffith et al., 2007). It is estimated that 9 to 21% of the *M. simiae* isolates from pulmonary specimens have clinical relevance (Rynkiewicz et al. 1998). The findings of this study suggest that members of this group may have pathogenic potential, but further studies are required to assess the characteristics of these isolates, including details on predisposing conditions from patients, as well as the drug susceptibility these NTM.

## 5. Conclusion

In conclusion, although our study is not necessarily representative for the whole Amazon region, it clearly demonstrates the importance of NTM pulmonary infections in this region. Our data also show that a variety of NTM species are involved, and that there is need for bacteriologic diagnosis in patients with TB, especially in patients who have failed TB treatment. We have shown that the lack of species identification in a significant subset (8.0%) of patients with a presumptive diagnosis of TB in a regional reference center can lead to misdiagnosis and may be followed by inadequate treatment.

## 6. Acknowledgment

This work was supported by the Fundação de Amparo à Pesquisa do Estado do Pará, the Coordenação de Aperfeiçoamento de Pessoal de Nível Superior, the Conselho Nacional de Desenvolvimento Científico e Tecnológico and the Evandro Chagas Institute, Ananindeua, Pará, Brazil.

## 7. References

Adékambi T, Drancourt M (2004) Dissection of phylogenetic relationships among 19 rapidly growing *Mycobacterium* species by 16S rRNA, *hsp65, sodA, recA* and *rpoB* gene sequencing. *Int J Syst Evol Microbiol* 54(Pt 6):2095-105. ISSN 1466-5034.

American Thoracic Society (1997) Diagnosis and treatment of disease caused by nontuberculous mycobacteria. This official statement of the American Thoracic Society was approved by the Board of Directors, March 1997. Medical Section of the American Lung Association. *Am J Respir Crit Care Med* 156(2 Pt 2):S1-25. ISSN 1073-449X.

Barreto AMW, Campos CED (2000) Micobactérias não-tuberculosas no Brasil. *Bol Pneum Sanit* 8(1):23-32. ISSN 0103-460X.

Billinger ME, Olivier KN, Viboud C, de Oca RM, Steiner C, Holland SM, Prevots DR (2009) Non tuberculosis mycobacteria associated lung disease in hospitalized persons in unites states 1998-2005. Emerg Infect Dis 2009; 15(10): 1562-1569.

Blackwood KS, He C, Gunton J, Turenne CY, Wolfe J, Kabani AM (2000) Evaluation of *recA* sequences for identification of *Mycobacterium* species. *J Clin Microbiol* 38(8):2846-2852. ISSN 1098-660X.

Bodle EE, Cunningham JA, Della-Latta P, Schluger NW, Saiman L (2008) Epidemiology of Nontuberculous Mycobacteria in Patients Without HIV Infection, New York City. *Emerg Infect Dis* 14(3):390-396. ISSN 1080-6059.

Brasil (2005) *Tuberculose: guia de vigilância epidemiológica.* 6th ed. Brasília: Ministério da Saúde, pp. 732–756. Retrieved from
http://bvsms.saude. gov/bvs/publicacoes/Guia_Vig_Epid_novo2.pdf

Brasil (2008) *Manual Nacional de Vigilância Laboratorial da Tuberculose e outras Micobactérias. Série A. Normas e Manuais Técnicos.* Brasília: Ministério da Saúde, Secretaria de Vigilância em Saúde 2008; pp.1-436. Retrieved from
http://portal.saude.gov.br/portal/arquivos/pdf/manual_laboratorio_tb.pdf.(a)

British Thoracic Society (2000) Management of opportunist mycobacterial infections: Joint Tuberculosis Committee Guidelines 1999. Subcommittee of the Joint Tuberculosis Committee of the British Thoracic Society. *Thorax* 55:210-218. ISSN 1468-3296.

Brown-Elliott BA, Wallace RJ Jr (2002) Clinical and taxonomic status of pathogenic nonpigmented or late-pigmenting rapidly growing mycobacteria. *Clin Microbiol Rev* 15(4):716-46. ISSN 0983-8512.

Cassidy PM, Hedberg K, Saulson A, McNelly E, Winthrop KL (2009) Nontuberculous mycobacterial disease prevalence and risk factors: a changing epidemiology. *Clin Infect Dis* 15;49(12):e124-9. ISSN 1058-4838.

Chan ED, Iseman MD (2010) Slender, older women appear to be more susceptible to nontuberculous mycobacterial lung disease. *Gend Med* 7(1):5-18.

da Costa ARF, Lopes ML, Bahia JRC, Conceição EC, Lima KVB (2010a) Identificação genotípica de membros do complexo *Mycobacterium avium* isolados de infecções pulmonares no Estado do Pará, Brasil. *Rev Pan-Amaz Saude* 1(3):35-42. ISSN 2176-6223.

da Costa ARF, Lopes ML, Furlaneto IP, Sousa MS, Lima KVB (2010b) Molecular identification of nontuberculous mycobacteria isolates in a Brazilian mycobacteria reference laboratory. *Diagn Microbiol Infect Dis* 68(4):390-394. ISSN 0732-8893.

da Costa ARF, Lopes ML, Leão SC, Schneider MPC, Sousa MS, Suffys PN, Corvelo TCO, Lima KVB (2009) Molecular identification of rapidly growing mycobacteria isolates from pulmonary specimens of patients in the State of Pará, Amazon region, Brazil. *Diagn Microbiol Infect Dis* 65(4):358-364. ISSN 0732-8893.

Di Lonardo M, Isola NC, Ambroggi M, Rybko A, Poggi S (1995) Mycobacteria in HIV-infected patients in Buenos Aires. *Tuber Lung Dis* 76(3):185-189. ISSN 0962-8479.

Domenech P, Menendez MC, Garcia MJ (1994) Restriction fragment length polymorphisms of 16S rRNA genes in the differentiation of fast-growing mycobacterial species. *FEMS Microbiol Let* 116(1):19-24. ISSN 0378-1097.

Euzéby JP (1997) List of bacterial names with standing in nomenclature: a folder available on the Internet. *Int J Syst Bacteriol* 47:590–592 List of prokaryotic names with standing in nomenclature. Last full update: July 09, 2011. URL: http://www.bacterio.cict.fr/m/mycobacterium.html.

Falkinham JO 3rd (2002) Nontuberculous mycobacteria in the environment. *Clin Chest Med* 23:529-551. ISSN 1557-8216

Falkinham JO 3rd (2009) Surrounded by mycobacteria: nontuberculous mycobacteria in the human environment. *J Appl Microbiol*107:356-367. ISSN 1364-5072.

Freeman J, Morris A, Blackmore T, Hammer D, Munroe S, McKnight L (2007) Incidence of nontuberculous mycobacterial disease in New Zealand, 2004. *N Z Med J.* 15;120(1256):U2580. ISSN 0028-8446.

Glassroth J (2008) Pulmonary disease due to nontuberculous mycobacteria. *Chest* 133(1):243-251. ISSN 0012-3692.

Good RC (1980) From the Center for Disease Control. Isolation of nontuberculous mycobacteria in the United States, 1979. *J Infect Dis* 142:779-783. ISSN 1537-6613.

Gopinath K, Singh S (2010) Non-tuberculous mycobacteria in TB-endemic countries: are we neglecting the danger? *PLoS Negl Trop Dis* 4:e615, doi:10.1371/journal.pntd.0000615. ISSN 1935-2735.

Griffith DE (2010) Nontuberculous mycobacterial lung disease. *Curr Opin Infect Dis* 23(2):185–190. ISSN 1473-6527.

Griffith DE, Aksamit T, Brown-Elliott BA, Catanzaro A, Daley C, Gordin F, Holland SM, Horsburgh R, Huitt G, Iademarco MF, Iseman M, Olivier K, Ruoss S, Fordham von Reyn C, Wallace Jr RJ, Winthrop K. American Thoracic Society (2007) An Official ATS/IDSA Statement: Diagnosis, Treatment, and Prevention of Nontuberculous Mycobactecterial Diseases. *Am J Respir Crit Care Med* 175:367-416. ISSN 1073-449X.

Griffith DE, Girard WM, Wallace RJ Jr (1993) Clinical features of pulmonary disease caused by rapidly growing mycobacteria. An analysis of 154 patients. *Am Rev Respir Dis* 147(5):1271-1278. ISSN 0003-0805.

Griffith DE (2007) Impact of new American Thoracic Society diagnostic criteria on management of nontuberculous mycobacterial infection. *Am J Respir Crit Care Med* 176:419. ISSN 1073-449X.

Iseman MD, Marras TK (2008) The importance of nontuberculous mycobacterial lung disease. *Am J Respir Crit Care Med.* 2008 15;178(10):999-1000. ISSN 1073-449X.

Jarzembowski JA, Young MB (2008) Nontuberculous mycobacterial infections. *Arch Pathol Lab Med* 132(8):1333-1341. ISSN 1543-2165.

Jeong YJ, Lee KS, Koh WJ, Han J, Kim TS, Kwon OJ (2004) Nontuberculous mycobacterial pulmonary infection in immunocompetent patients: comparison of thin-section CT and histopathologic findings. *Radiology* 231(3):880-886. ISSN 1527- 1315.

Katoch VM (2004) Infections due to non-tuberculous mycobacteria (NTM). *Indian J Med Res* 120(4):290-304. ISSN 0971-5916.

Kendall BA, Varley CD, Choi D, Cassidy PM, Hedberg K, Ware MA, Winthrop KL (2011) Distinguishing tuberculosis from nontuberculous mycobacteria lung disease, Oregon, USA. *Emerg Infect Dis* 17(3):506-9. ISSN 1080-6059.

Kim H, Kim SH, Shim TS, Kim M, Bai GH, Park YG, Lee SH, Chae GT, Cha CY, Kook YH, Kim BJ (2005) Differentiation of *Mycobacterium* species by analysis of the heat-shock protein 65 gene (*hsp65*). *Int J Syst Evol Microbiol* 55:1649–1656. ISSN 1466-5034.

Kobashi Y, Matsushima T (2007) The microbiological and clinical effects of combined therapy according to guidelines on the treatment of pulmonary *Mycobacterium avium* complex disease in Japan - including a follow-up study. *Respiration* 74:394–400. ISSN 1423-0356.

Koh WJ, Kwon OJ, Lee KS (2005) Diagnosis and treatment of nontuberculous mycobacterial pulmonary diseases: a Korean perspective. *J Korean Med Sci* 20:913–925. ISSN 1011-8934.

Kubica GP (1973) Differential identification of mycobacteria. *Am Rev Resp Dis* 107: 9-12. ISSN: 0003-0805.

Lee H, Park HJ, Cho SN, Bai GH, Kim SJ (2000) Species identification of mycobacteria by PCR-restriction fragment length polymorphism of the *rpoB* gene. *J Clin Microbiol* 38(8):2966-2971. ISSN 1098-660X.

León CI (1998) Presencia de las micobacterias no tuberculosas en Colombia. *Médicas UIS* 12: 181-187. ISSN 1794-5240.

Marras TK, Chedore P; Ying AM, Jamieson F (2007) Isolation prevalence of pulmonary non-tuberculous mycobacteria in Ontario, 1997–2003. *Thorax* 62:661-666. ISSN 1468-3296.

Marras TK, Daley CL (2002) Epidemiology of human pulmonary infection with nontuberculous mycobacteria. *Clin Chest Med* 23:553–567. ISSN 1557-8216.

Martin A, Uwizeye C, Fissette K, De Rijk P, Palomino JC, Leão S, Portaels PC, Scarparo C (2009) Extrapulmonary infections associated with nontuberculous mycobacteria in immunocompetent persons. *Emerg Infect Dis* 15:1351–1358. ISSN 1080-6059.

Parrish SC, Myers J, Lazarus A (2008) Nontuberculous mycobacterial pulmonary infections in Non-HIV patients. *Postgrad Med* 120(4):78-86. ISSN 0032-5481.

Pedro HSP, Pereira MIF, Goloni MRA, Ueki SYM, Chimara E (2008) Isolamento de micobactérias não-tuberculosas em São José do Rio Preto entre 1996 e 2005. *J Bras Pneumol* 34(11):950-955. ISSN 1806-3713.

Prevots DR, Shaw PA, Strickland D, Jackson LA, Raebel MA, Blosky MA, Montes de Oca R, Shea YR, Seitz AE, Holland SM, Olivier KN (2010) Nontuberculous mycobacterial lung disease prevalence at four integrated healthcare delivery systems. *AM J Respir Crit Care Med* 182:970-976. ISSN 1073-449X.

Reich JM, Johnson RE (1995) Mycobacterium avium complex lung disease in women. *Chest* 107(1):293-295. ISSN 1931-3543.

Roth A, Fischer M, Hamid ME, Michalke S, Ludwig W, Mauch H (1998) Differentiation of phylogenetically related slowly growing mycobacteria based on 16S-23S rRNA gene internal transcribed spacer sequences. *J Clin Microbiol* 36(1):139-147. ISSN 1098-660X.

Runyon EH (1959) Anonymous mycobacteria in pulmonary disease. *Med Clin North Am.* 43(1):273-290. ISSN 1557-9859.

Rynkiewicz DL, Cage GD, Butler WR, Ampel NM (1998) Clinical and microbiological assessment of *Mycobacterium simiae* isolates from a single laboratory in southern Arizona. *Clin Infect Dis* 26(3):625-30. ISSN 1058-4838.

Santos RMC, Ogusku MM, Miranda JM, Dos Santos MC, Salem JI (2006) Avaliação da reação em cadeia da polimerase no diagnóstico da tuberculose pulmonar em pacientes indígenas e não indígenas. *J Bras Pneumol* 32(3):234-240. ISSN 1806-3713.

Sexton P, Harrison AC (2008) Susceptibility to nontuberculous mycobacterial lung disease. *Eur Respir J* 31: 1322–1333. ISSN 1399-3003.

Shin S, Kim EC, Yoon JH (2006) Identification of nontuberculous mycobacteria by sequence analysis of the 16S ribosomal RNA, the heat shock protein 65 and the RNA polymerase β-subunit genes. *Korean J Lab Med* 26:153–160. ISSN 1598-6535.

Shin JH, Cho EJ, Lee JY, Yu JY, Kang YH (2009) Novel diagnostic algorithm using *tuf* gene amplification and restriction fragment length polymorphism is promising tool for identification of nontuberculous mycobacteria. *J Microbiol Biotechnol* 19(3):323-330. ISSN 1017-7825.

Simons S, van Ingen J, Hsueh PR, Van Hung N, Dekhuijzen PN, Boeree MJ, van Soolingen D (2011) Nontuberculous mycobacteria in respiratory tract infections, eastern Asia. *Emerg Infect Dis* 17(3):343-349. ISSN 1080-6059.

Takewaki S, Okuzumi K, Manabe I, Tanimura M, Miyamura K, Nakahara K, Yazaki Y, Ohkubo A, Nagai R (1994) Nucleotide sequence comparison of the mycobacterial *dnaJ* gene and PCR-restriction fragment length polymorphism analysis for identification of mycobacterial species. *Int J Syst Bacteriol* 44(1):159-166. ISSN 0020-7713.

Telenti A, Marchesi F, Balz M, Bally F, Böttger EC, Bodmer T (1993) Rapid identification of mycobacteria to the species level by polymerase chain reaction and restriction enzyme analysis. *J Clin Microbiol* 31:175–178. ISSN 1098-660X.

Tortoli E (2003) Impact of genotypic studies on mycobacterial taxonomy: the new mycobacteria of the 1990s. *Clin Microbiol Rev* 16:319–354. ISSN 1098-6618.

Tortoli E (2006) The new mycobacteria: an update. *FEMS Immunol Med Microbiol* 48(2):159-178. ISSN 1574-695X.

Tortoli E (2009) Clinical manifestations of nontuberculous mycobacteria infections. *Clin Microbiol Infect* 15(10):906-10. ISSN 1469-0691.

Tortoli E, Böttger EC, Fabio A, Falsen E, Gitti Z, Grottola A, Klenk HP, Mannino R, Mariottini A, Messinò M, Pecorari M, Rumpianesi F (2010) *Mycobacterium europaeum* sp. nov., a scotochromogenic species related to *Mycobacterium simiae* complex. *Int J Syst Evol Microbiol.* ijs.0.025601-0v1-ijs.0.025601-0. ISSN 1466-5034.

Tortoli E, Rindi L, Garcia MJ, Chiaradonna P, Dei R, Garzelli C, et al (2004) Proposal to elevate the genetic variant MAC-A, included in the *Mycobacterium avium* complex, to species rank as *Mycobacterium chimaera* sp. nov. *Int J Syst Evol Microbiol* 54:1277-1285. ISSN 1466-5034.

Tsukamura M, Kita N, Shimoide H, Arakawa H, Kuze A (1988). Studies on the epidemiology of nontuberculous mycobacteriosis in Japan. *Am Rev Respir Dis* 137: 1280-1284. ISSN 0003-0805.

Ueki SYM, Telles MAS, Virgilio MC, Giampaglia CMS, Chimara E, Ferrazoli L (2005) Micobactérias não-tuberculosas: diversidade das espécies no estado de São Paulo. *J Bras Patol Med Lab* 41(1):1-8. ISSN 1676- 2444.

van Ingen J, Bendien SA, de Lange WC, Hoefsloot W, Dekhuijzen PN, Boeree MJ, van Soolingen D (2009) Clinical relevance of non-tuberculous mycobacteria isolated in the Nijmegen-Arnhem region, The Netherlands. *Thorax* 64:502–506. ISSN 1468-3296.

van Ingen J, Boeree MJ, de Lange WC, Dekhuijzen PN, van Soolingen D (2007) Impact of new American Thoracic Society diagnostic criteria on management of nontuberculous mycobacterial infection. *Am J Respir Crit Care Med* 176:418-419. ISSN 1073-449X

von Reyn CF, Waddell RD, Eaton T, Arbeit RD, Maslow JN, Barber TW, Brindle RJ, Gilks CF, Lumio J, Lähdevirta J, Ranki A, Dawson D, Falkinham JO 3rd (1993) Isolation of *Mycobacterium avium* complex from water in the United States, Finland, Zaire, and Kenya. *J Clin Microbiol* 1993;12:3227-3230. ISSN 1098-660X.

Wallace RJ Jr (1994) *Mycobacterium avium* complex lung disease and women. Now an equal opportunity disease. *Chest* 105(1):6-7. ISSN 1931-3543.

Webb, WR (1962) Clinical evaluation of a new mucolytic agent, acetylcysteine. *J. Thoracic Cardiovascular Surg.* 44:330-343. ISSN: 0022-5223.

Whipps CM, Butler WR, Pourahmad F, Watral VG, Kent ML (2007) Molecular systematics support the revival of *Mycobacterium salmoniphilum* (ex Ross 1960) sp. nov., nom. rev., a species closely related to *Mycobacterium chelonae*. *Int J Syst Evol Microbiol* 57(Pt 11):2525-31. ISSN 1466-5034.

Winthrop KL, McNelley E, Kendall B, Marshall-Olson A, Morris C, Cassidy M, Saulson A, Hedberg K (2010) Pulmonary nontuberculous mycobacterial disease prevalence and clinical features: an emerging public health disease. *Am J Respir Crit Care Med* 1;182(7):977-82. ISSN 1073-449X.

Zamarioli LA, Coelho AGV, Pereira CM, Nascimento ACC, Ueki SYM, Chimara E (2008) Descriptive study of the frequency of nontuberculous mycobacteria in the Baixada Santista region of the state of São Paulo, Brazil. *J Bras Pneumol* 34(8):590-594. ISSN 1806-3713.

# 4

# Nontuberculous Mycobacterial Pulmonary Disease

Ante Marušić[1] and Mateja Janković[2]
[1]*Poliklinika "Medikol", Department of Radiology*
[2]*University Medical Centre Zagreb,*
*University Hospital for Lung Diseases "Jordanovac"*
*Croatia*

## 1. Introduction

Tuberculosis (TB) is an infectious and transmissible disease caused by *Mycobacterium tuberculosis* and closely related mycobacterial species (*M. bovis, M. africanum,* and *M. microti*). These species, obligate pathogens, compose what is known as the *M. tuberculosis complex*. Nontuberculous mycobacterial (NTM) species are mycobacterial species other than those belonging to the *Mycobacterium tuberculosis complex*. Nontuberculous mycobacteria are generally free-living organisms that are ubiquitous in the environment. There have been more than 140 NTM species identified. In 1959, Runyon proposed a classification of NTM into four major groups, based on growth rate and colony pigmentation (Runyon EH , 1959).

There is an increasing number of clinical isolates of NTM in many countries and growing awareness of their ability to cause disease (American Thoracic Society [ATS], 2007). Nontuberculous mycobacteria are capable of causing a wide range of infections in humans with pulmonary NTM disease being the most common, especially in patients with pre-existent pulmonary disease (ATS, 2007). They are mainly opportunistic pathogens that can occasionally cause severe disseminated diseases, especially in patients with systemic impairment of immunity. Identification of specific species of NTM is important because of the variation in antimicrobial susceptibility and treatment options.

Nontuberculous mycobacteria can be divided into slowly growing and rapidly growing mycobacteria (RGM). The former constitute members of the Runyon group I to group III, whereas the latter are equivalent to the members of Runyon group IV. (Table 1) (Runyon E, 1965) Pulmonary disease is primarily caused by *M. avium complex (MAC)* and *M. kansasii (*ATS, 2007*)*. Other species include *M. abscessus, M. fortuitum, M. xenopi, M. malmoense, M. szulgai,* and *M. simiae*. In contrast to *M. tuberculosis,* isolation of NTM does not necessarily mean that patient has the disease though it can be isolated transiently from respiratory specimens. In order to assist clinicians with the difficult task of trying to determine if a given NTM species is causing disease to a patient, a set of criteria utilizing clinical, radiographic, and microbiologic parameters has been developed. Furthermore, the degree of evidence to support the choice of treatment is limited because a few clinical trials have been conducted, especially for disease due to less prevalent NTM species.

| |
|---|
| *Mycobacterium tuberculosis* complex |
| *M. tuberculosis* |
| *M. bovis* |
| *M. africanum* |
| *M. microti* |
| Slowly growing mycobacteria |
| Runyon Group I, Photochromogenes |
| *M. kansasii* |
| *M. marinum* |
| Runyon Group II, Scotochromogenes |
| *M. gordonae* |
| *M. scrofulaceum* |
| Runyon Group III, Non-chromogenes |
| *M. avium complex – M. avium, M. intracellulare* |
| *M. terrae complex* |
| *M. ulcerans* |
| *M. xenopi* |
| *M. simiae* |
| *M. malmoense* |
| *M. szulgai* |
| *M. asiaticum* |
| Rapidly growing mycobacteria |
| Runyon group IV |
| *M. fortuitum* |
| *M. chelonae* |
| *M. abscesus* |

Table 1. Classification of mycobacterial species commonly causing human disease

Current guidelines are mainly based on case reports and clinical experience (ATS 2007, British thoracic society [BTS], 1999)

## 2. Epidemiology and prevalence

Tuberculosis still remains an important public health problem worldwide, with more than 9 million new cases of tuberculosis reported every year and decrease of incidence of less than 1% per year. On the other hand, in the industrialized world, the incidence of *M. tuberculosis* infections has been decreasing, while the incidence of NTM pulmonary infections is increasing.

Although both *M. tuberculosis* and NTM cause chronic lung infections, only *M. tuberculosis* spreads from person to person by inhalation of organisms expectorated into the air. Nontuberculous mycobacteria infections are not considered contagious. Since reporting NTM pulmonary disease to public health departments is not obligatory, the exact number of the infected remains unknown. An increase in the frequency of NTM infections and NTM pulmonary disease has been indicated in a number of worldwide surveys and population-based studies during the last few decades (AST, 2007; Maras et al, 2007; Iseman & Marras, 2008; Henry et al, 2004; Thomson & Yew, 2009).

Postulated reasons for this increase include a rise in prevalence of HIV infections and other acquired immunocompromised states, increased awareness of these organisms as potential pathogens, a better understanding of clinical-pathological relationship between host and pathogen, advances in methods of detection of the organisms, an aging population (as this is often a disease of the elderly), increased survival of patients with predisposing conditions such as cystic fibrosis and COPD, and increased environmental exposure (ATS, 2007; Thomson & Yew, 2009).

Nontuberculous mycobacteria disease is not a reportable condition in most countries because it is not considered a public health concern on account of unknown or non-existing evidence of human-to-human transmission (ATS, 2007). However, the organisms are ubiquitous in the environment, oligotrophic and many NTM pathogens have been isolated from potable water where they can be found forming biofilms (Falkingham et al, 2001). *Mycobacterium avium* complex (MAC), *Mycobacterium kansasii* and RGM such as *M. abscessus* and *M. fortuitum* constitute the main species associated with human pulmonary disease. (ATS, 2007; Thomsen et al, 2002; Martin-Casabona et al, 2004). It has been shown in multiple already published studies that geography has a prominent role in the epidemiology of NTM pulmonary disease. Thus, *M. xenopi* is relatively more common in the south-east and in the west of Europe (Marusic et al, 2009; van Ingen et al, 2008; Hanry et al, 2004; Dailloux et al, 2006) and in Canada (Varadi & Marras, 2009), while *M. malmoense* is relatively more common in the north of Europe (Abgueguen et al, 2010; Petrini, 2006; Thomsen et al, 2002; Henry et al, 2004).

## 3. Pulmonary disease characteristics and population at risk

The symptoms of NTM pulmonary disease are variable and nonspecific. Common symptoms are chronic or recurring cough, while others such as sputum production, fatigue, malaise, dyspnea, fever, hemoptysis and weight loss become more prevalent with advanced NTM lung disease.

Pulmonary NTM disease has three distinct presentations: cavitary disease (resembling conventional tuberculosis) (Figure 1) (Moore, 1993; Patz et al, 1995; Jeong et al, 2004), nodular-bronchiectatic disease (Figure 2) commonly affecting the right middle lobe and lingula (Moore, 1993; Patz et al, 1995; Jeong et al 2004; Reich & Johnson, 1992) and the rarest form - hypersensitivity pneumonitis. There are mixed disease forms with infiltrates, nodes, bronchiectasis and interstitial changes (Figure 3).

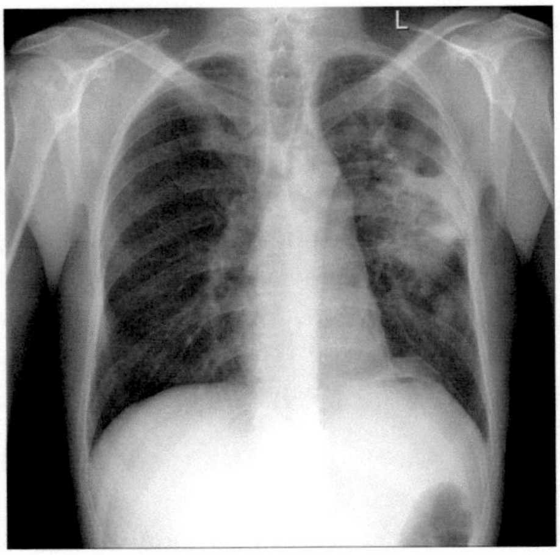


Fig. 1. Extensive infiltrate with cavitation in the left lung

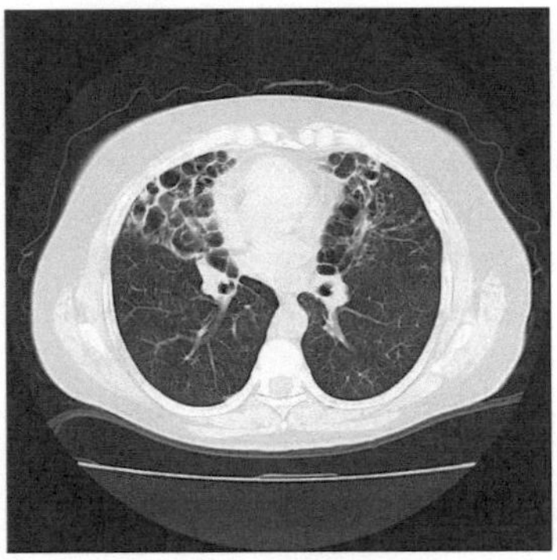

Fig. 2. Nodular-bronchiectatic disease in the middle lobe and lingula

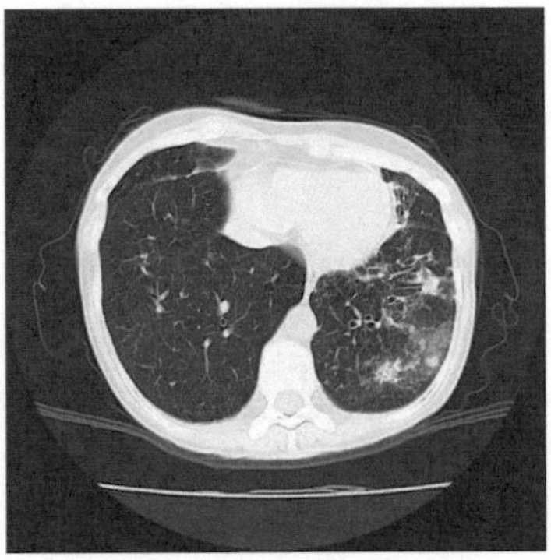

Fig. 3. Mixed disease form; infiltrate, nodes, bronchiectasis, "ground glass" interstitial pattern and tiny centrilobular nodes in left lower lobe

HIV-positive and other immunodeficient patients, on the other hand, often have hilar and mediastinal lymphadenopathy with systemic spread but without pulmonary infiltrate (dos Santos et al, 2008). Patients with NTM pulmonary disease often have predisposing structural lung disease, i.e. chronic obstructive pulmonary disease, cystic fibrosis, bronchiectasis, pneumoconiosis, prior tuberculosis, alveolar proteinosis, or chronic aspiration (ATS, 2007; Field & Cowie, 2006).

Among women with pulmonary disease, there is often constellation of physical findings such as bronchiectasis, thin body habitus and mitral valve prolapse (Prince et al, 1989; Kim et al, 2008). The reason for this association has not been determined and no significant immunological abnormality has been identified.

## 4. Diagnosis of NTM pulmonary infections

Patients seeking treatment who have respiratory samples positive for acid-fast bacilli (AFB) present a public health dilemma. Although Mycobacterium tuberculosis and NTM cause chronic lung infections, only tuberculosis (TB) spreads from person to person by inhalation of organisms expectorated into the air, while NTM infections are acquired directly from the environment. Diagnosing mycobacterial infections is often quite a challenge. Under the microscope, NTM and *M. tuberculosis* appear similar. Careful laboratory investigations must be performed to differentiate them. The definitive identification of mycobacterial species, which can take several weeks, and the inability to quickly distinguish NTM from TB on clinical grounds makes it difficult for public health officials to make decisions regarding contact investigations and isolation. Mycobacterial pulmonary disease usually progresses slowly, and clinical diagnosis starts with the exclusion of other possible causes. Differential diagnosis includes tuberculosis and fungal infection, especially the classical form of NTM infection which mimics *M. tuberculosis* infection. The development and use of molecular techniques to differentiate between the mycobacteria strains made it possible to solve some of these problems. The first step in diagnosing an NTM infection is suspecting an underlying cause of the symptoms or radiographic findings. Chronic cough (lasting >3 weeks), fatigue, night sweats, and weight loss should make clinicians consider mycobacterial infections. Even though dyspnoea is usually more related to underlying lung disease, occasionally patients with the nodular/bronchiectatic disease can have bronchiolitis and air trapping associated with dyspnoea. Haemoptysis occurs in more advanced lung disease, especially with cavitations and advanced bronchiectasis. A chest radiograph, or more likely, high resolution computed tomography (HRCT), could show some radiomorphologic changes to be the first sign of presence of an NTM infection. Respiratory specimens should be obtained and sent for mycobacterial culture.

### 4.1 Imaging of NTM pulmonary infections

A chest radiograph is the first method to be used when suspecting an NTM pulmonary disease but it may be adequate for evaluating only patients with fibrocavitary disease. It is widely available and convenient and exposes patient to a very low irradiation dose. On the other hand, chest radiograph is far less sensitive and specific than HRCT, especially in detection of bronchiectasis, small nodules and other interstitial lung changes. Since nodular/bronchiectatic form of pulmonary NTM infection is not rare, HRCT should be used in patients with high clinical suspicion even if chest x-ray finding is normal. In case of clinical suspicion of hypersensitivity pneumonitis, HRCT is definitively the only method of choice. Even though some differences have been reported, it is impossible to differentiate

NTM pulmonary disease from TB pulmonary disease relying on radiographic appearance alone. Compared with radiographic findings in TB, patients with NTM disease and predominantly fibrocavitary radiographic changes tend to have following characteristics: thin-walled cavities with less surrounding parenchymal opacity, more contiguous spread of disease, and production of more marked involvement of pleura over the involved area of the lungs (ATS, 2007). Basal pleural disease is not often found and pleural effusion is rare (ATS, 2007). At patients with predominantly nodular/bronchiectatic disease, the abnormalities on chest radiograph and HRCT are primarily found in the mid and lower lung field. Radiographic follow-up during the treatment should be performed using either chest radiograph in patients with predominantly cavitary disease, or HRCT in those with interstitial form of the disease. Confirmation of complete resolution and an insight into possible residual scarring can be done only by using HRCT.

### 4.2 Laboratory features of NTM

Using modern microbiology laboratory methods, including liquid culture media, NTM growth can be detected by culture from a patient's specimens 1-3 weeks after the incubation. (Leitritz et al, 2001) Most rapid growing NTM will grow in 7-10 days. Slow growers can grow in 1-3 weeks, but may take much longer. Therefore, cultures are usually kept for 6-8 weeks before being regarded as negative. At patients colonized with *Pseudomonas aeruginosa* or other bacterial pathogens, sputum specimens can be overgrown before NTM growth appears. Special decontamination methods are often necessary to reduce this overgrowth, but decontamination also reduces the yield of mycobacteria and persistence is required if there is a high clinical suspicion of NTM disease with these patients. With the recovery of an organism by culture, DNA probes are commercially available to identify some of the NTM (Tortoli et al, 2010).

Other organisms have traditionally been identified by combination of biochemical testing, high-performance liquid chromatography (HPLC) and genetic sequencing of conserved regions. Partial sequencing of a segment of 16S ribosomal RNA has been used to identify those species not identified by other means. (Cloud et al, 2002, 2005) Current guidelines of American Thoracic Society/Infectious Diseases Society of America (ATS/IDSA) (ATS, 2007) state that routine testing of MAC species for antimicrobial susceptibility (other than clarithromycin) is generally not recommended because of the paucity evidence correlating *in vitro* and *in vivo* results (ATS, 2007). They do recommend clarithromycin susceptibility testing for new, previously untreated MAC isolates as macrolide resistance has been associated with a poorer outcome. It should also be performed for MAC isolates from patients who have relapsed from apparently successful treatment or those who have failed macrolide treatment (ATS, 2007). Previously untreated *M. kansasii* strains should be tested *in vitro* to rimfapicin only (ATS 2007) and against a panel of secondary agents if shown to be resistant to rimfapicin. RGM should be tested against a panel of eight antimicrobials, including clarithromycin, amikacin, cefoxitin, ciprofloxacin, doxycicline, linezolid, sulphamethoxazole and tobramycin.

### 4.3 Diagnostic criteria

Even after an NTM has been isolated and identified, the patient may still not have the disease because NTM can be isolated transiently from respiratory specimens. In order to help clinicians with the difficult task of trying to determine if a given NTM species is causing disease in a patient the ATS/IDSA developed a set of criteria that utilized clinical, radiographic, and microbiologic parameters (ATS, 2007) (Table 2).

| |
|---|
| Clinical criteria<br>Compatible respiratory symptoms<br>Appropriate exclusion of other diagnoses, especially tuberculosis and mycosis |
| AND |
| Radiographic criteria<br>Nodular or cavity opacities on chest radiograph, or<br>a HRCT scan that shows multifocal bronchiectasis with or without<br>multiple small nodules |
| AND |
| Microbiological criteria |
| Positive culture results from at least two or three separately expectorated<br>sputum samples with positive or negative AFB smear, respectively |
| OR |
| Positive culture results from at least one bronchial wash or lavage |
| OR |
| Transbronchial or other lung biopsy with mycobacterial histopatological<br>features and one positive sputum culture for NTM |

Table 2. Summary of the ATS/IDSA criteria for diagnosis of pulmonary NTM diseases

The significance of an isolate also varies with the species of mycobacteria. Isolation of mycobacteria like *M. gordonae, M. flavescens, M. terrae complex* or *M. triviale* usually indicates transient colonization or possible contamination of the sample. However, *M. szulgai* is rarely isolated from the environment and a single positive culture provides pathological significance (ATS, 2007).

## 5. Treatment and prognosis of NTM pulmonary infections

The currently used regimen for TB treatment consists of four drugs: rifampin (RIF), isoniazid (INH), pyrazinamide (PZA), and ethambutol (EMB), for the duration of six to nine months. Treatment of pulmonary NTM infections is usually more complicated than treatment of tuberculosis. Drugs, administration frequency, and duration of therapy will vary depending on species of NTM causing the disease, extent and the site of infection. Some antituberculosis drugs are also active against some NTM species. However, treatment of most NTM species also requires administration of antibiotics that are not typically used to treat tuberculosis. The prognosis for NTM pulmonary disease depends on specific species and subspecies involved and their drugs susceptibility pattern, presence of other medical problems and whether or not patient can tolerate the treatment regimen. Cure rate for the disease caused by *M. kansasii* is similar to *M. tuberculosis* round 90%, while that for the disease caused by *M. avium* is 30-85%. Complete recovery is seldom achieved in patients with pulmonary *M. abscessus* infection (ATS, 2007).

Diagnosing pulmonary NTM infection/disease does not equate the need for immediate treatment since treatment usually involves combination antibiotic therapy for 12-24 months and constitutes an important undertaking for the patient. Lung involvement may range in severity from mild clinical (indolent) infection to disease associated with extensive invasion or destruction of the lungs. In some cases the disease remits spontaneously. Most of the early studies on NTM covered MAC, *M. kansasii* and *M. abscessus* and developed diagnostic criteria and treatment regimens best suitable for these species. There is not enough knowledge about most other NTM to be certain that the diagnostic criteria are universally applicable for all NTM respiratory pathogens (ATS, 2007). Generally, patients respond best to NTM treatment first time it is administered. Therefore, it is important that patients initially receive a recommended multi-drug regimen (ATS, 2007).

The British Thoracic Society (BTS) and ATS/IDSA have published guidelines for the management of the disease caused by NTM. Guidelines published by ATS/IDSA have been updated in 2007 providing an extensive review of the available literature on NTM disease combined with expert opinion. The recommended criteria are thus based on several smaller prospective non-randomized controlled studies at the US patients.

It is very difficult to compare many different studies in pulmonary NTM disease considering the geographic differences in patient populations, mixture of disease types, severity of disease, differing species of NTM, drugs and therapy protocols used and different study design and analysis. The BTS guidelines are predominantly based on two large randomized controlled trials performed in patients of the UK and Europe (BTS, 2001). All of the mentioned differences are factors contributing to the significant heterogeneity of findings and hence the recommendations made by the Societies.

Treatment of pulmonary disease should be considered in patients who meet clinical, radiological, and microbiologic criteria for NTM disease. Two main factors to consider regarding initiation of therapy should be pathogenicity of species and rate of disease progression. Therapy for NTM requires prolonged administration of multiple drugs and is associated with significant side effects. The decision to institute treatment in patients with non-cavitary disease who do not have clearly progressive pulmonary disease should be made carefully, after a period of clinical and radiological follow-up. The aim of therapy is a 12-month period of negative sputum cultures.

## 5.1 Specific antimicrobial treatment guidelines

### 5.1.1 MAC lung disease

Recommended treatment regimens for MAC lung disease are summarized in Table 3. There are still a number of controversies and unresolved questions regarding the management of MAC lung disease.

First, there is no demonstrated superiority of one macrolide among the two agents regarding efficacy or risk of resistance. It seems that macrolides have helped improving treatment of MAC lung disease (Kobashi YMT, 2004) though not all studies have supported this (Jenkins et al, 2008).

Second, there has also been no demonstrated superiority of one rifamycin (rifabutin or rifampicin) in the treatment of MAC lung disease, but because of frequent adverse events,

| | |
|---|---|
| Nodular/bronchiectatic disease | |
| All given 3 times weekly | Clarithromycin (1000 mg) or azithromycin (500 mg) + |
| | Rifampin (600 mg) + |
| | Ethambutol (25 mg/kg) |
| Fibrocavitary MAC lung disease or severe nodular/bronchiectatic disease | |
| All given daily | Clarithromycin (500–1000 mg) or azithromycin (250 mg) + |
| | Rifampin (600 mg) or rifabutin (150–300 mg) + |
| | Ethambutol (15 mg/kg) |
| | Consider adding 3-times-weekly amikacin or streptomycin early in therapy (e.g., for the first 8 weeks) |
| Duration: | Treat until cultures have been negative on therapy for 1 year. |

Table 3. Recommended treatment regimens for MAC pulmonary disease

most experts recommend the use of rifampicin (Griffith et al, 1995) Regarding the use of an amynoglicoside in the initial phase of treatment, the majority of early macrolides studies performed in the USA included 2- to 3-month period of intermittent amynoglicoside. Furthermore, Kobashi has shown that sputum conversion rates, relapse rates and overall outcomes were better in the cohort that received amynoglicoside (Kobashi YMT, 2004).

For hypersensitivity pneumonitis due to MAC, removal from environmental exposure is mandatory. Corticosteroids and/or anti-microbial drugs might be required in some cases and usually a shorter regimen of 3-6 months may be appropriate. (Hanak et al, 2006)

### 5.1.2 *M. kansasii* lung disease

Recommended treatment regimen for *M. kansasii* lung disease is summarized in Table 4. For susceptible strains, rifampin is the foundation of a multiple-drug regimen. Resistance to rifampin may develop, in which case a 3-drug regimen should be chosen on the basis of in vitro susceptibility testing (e.g., clarithromycin or azithromycin, moxifloxacin, ethambutol, sulphamethoxazole, or streptomycin) (ATS 2007).

### 5.1.3 *M. xenopi, M. malmoense* and *M. szulgai* lung disease

*M. xenopi* has variable drug susceptibility testing results, especially regarding the first-line antituberculotic agents (ATS, 2007). The clinical response to treatment does not always correlate well with drug susceptibility testing results. The ATS proposed regimen is a combination of ethambutol, rifampicin, isoniasid and clarithromycin with or without an initial course of streptomycin. *M. malmoense* can be difficult to treat. A combination of rifampicin and ethambutol with or without isoniasid has shown some effectiveness (BTS 2001). *M. szulgai* is susceptible in vitro to most antituberculosis drugs, as well as to floroquinolones and macrolides (Sanchez-Alarcos et al, 2003) and a 3- or 4-drug regimen that includes 12 months of negative sputum cultures while on therapy is recommended (ATS, 2007)

| | |
|---|---|
| Rifampin | 600 mg/d, + |
| Isoniazid | 300 mg/d, + |
| Ethambutol | 15 mg/kg/d |
| Duration: | at least 12 months after the last positive sputum culture |

Table 4. Recommended treatment regimens for rifampicin-susceptible *Mycobacterium kansasii* pulmonary disease

### 5.1.4 Lung disease caused by rapidly growing mycobacteria

Three main species of RGM causing pulmonary disease are *M. abscessus*, *M. chelonae* and *M. fortuitum*. The choice of treatment relies on guidance from susceptibility testing as there are no results from large-scale clinical studies available. *M. abscessus* pulmonary disease can be especially difficult to treat.

The treatment usually involves combination of amikacin, cefoxitin/imipenem and clarithromycin. The summary of proposed treatment for RGM lung disease is shown in Table 5. For many patients, realistic objectives of treatment are to help controlling symptoms and disease progression rather than curing the infection. Surgery can be considered for localized disease.

### 5.1.5 Surgical treatment

Surgical resection of limited (focal) pulmonary NTM disease in a patient with an adequate cardiopulmonary reserve can be successful in combination with multi-drug treatment regimens for MAC and *M. abscessus* disease (ATS, 2007). In addition, in an extensive disease, the excision of large cavitary mycobacterial foci might assist medical management of remaining lesions. However, according to ATS guidelines, surgery should only be performed in medical centres with considerable medical and surgical expertise in management of patients with NTM disease.

| | *Active drugs* | *Surgery* |
|---|---|---|
| *M. abscessus* | Clarithromycin | ++ |
| | Amikacin | |
| | Cefoxitin | |
| | Imipenem | |
| *M. chelonae* | Tobramycin | + |
| | Clarithromycin | |
| | Linezolid | |
| | Imipenem | |
| | Amikacin | |
| | Doxycycline | |
| | Ciprofloxacin | |
| *M. fortuitum* | Amikacin | + |
| | Ofloxacin/Ciprofloxacin | |
| | Imipenem | |
| | Sulphonamides | |
| | Clarithromycin | |
| | Doxycycline | |

Table 5. Treatment of lung disease due to rapidly growing mycobacteria

## 6. Where do we go from here?

Given the recent worldwide increase in NTM infections and in comparison to other lung diseases, relatively little progress has been made in understanding, preventing or treating pulmonary NTM disease. It is still not clear why some people develop infections while most do not. Even though information is provided from basic research and a few clinical trials, better understanding of the pathogenesis of these infections is needed in order to improve prevention of harm from these ubiquitous environmental bacteria. As NTM lung diseases are generally difficult to treat, new drugs are needed to advance therapy. Furthermore, randomized controlled trials in well-described patients would provide stronger evidence-based data to guide therapy of NTM lung diseases. Elucidation of the mechanism behind host susceptibility will also add invaluable information so that therapy could be directed towards the underlying cause for the establishment of infection. Finally, environmental factors contributing to the increased prevalence of infection should also be explored in order to reduce infection and re-infection of susceptible patients.

## 7. References

Abgueguen P, Rabier V, Mahaza C, Warot A, Chennebault JM, Pichard E. Mycobacterium malmoense: an underestimated nontuberculous mycobacterium. Diagn Microbiol Infect Dis. 2010; 66(1):98-100.

Cloud JL, Neal H, Rosenberry R, Turenne CY , Jama M et al. Identification of *Mycobacterium* spp. By using a comercial 16S ribosomal DNA sequecing kit and additional sequencing libraries. J Clin Microbiol 2002;40:400-6.

Cloud JL, Hoggan K, Belousov E, Cohen S, Brown-Elliott BA et al. Use of MGB eclipse system and SmartCycler PCR for differentiation of *Mycobacterium chelonae* and *M. abscessus*. J Clin Microbiol 2005; 43:4205-7.

Dailloux M, Abalain ML, Laurain C, Lebrun L, Loos-Ayav C, Lozniewski A Maugein J; French Mycobacteria Study Group. Respiratory infections associated with nontuberculous mycobacteria in non-HIV patients. Eur Respir J. 2006; 28(6):1211-5.

dos Santos RP, Scheid KL, Willers DM, Goldani LZ. Comparative radiological features of disseminated disease due to Mycobacterium tuberculosis vs. non-tuberculosis mycobacteria among AIDS patients in Brazil. BMC Infect Dis. 2008; 8:24.

Falkingham JO III, Norton CD, Le Cchavaillier MW. Factors influencing numbers of Mycobacterium avium, *Mycobacterium intracellulare*, and other mycobacteria in drinking water distribution systems. Appl Environ Microbiol. 2001;67:1225-31.

Field SK & Cowie RL. Lung disease due to the more common nontuberculous mycobacteria. Chest 2006; 129:1653-1672.

Griffith D, Brown-Elliott B, Girard W & Wallace R Jr. Adverse events associated with high-dose rifambutin in macrolide-containing regimens for treatment of Mycobacterium avium complex lung disease. Clin Infect Dis 1995;21:594-8.

Griffith DE, Aksamit T, Brown-Elliot BA, Catanzaro A, Daley C, Gordin F, Holland, SM, Horsburgh R, Huitt G, Iademarco MF, Iseman M, Olivier K, Ruoss S, von Reyn CF, Wallace RJ Jr, Winthrop K et al, for the ATS Mycobacterial Disease Subcommittee; American Thoracic Society; Infectious Disease Society of America. An official ATS/IDSA statement. Diagnosis, treatment, and prevention of Nontuberculous mycobacterial diseases. Am J Respir Crit Care Med 2007;175:367-416.

Hanak V, Kalra S, Aksamit TR, Hartman TE, Tazelaar HD et al. Hot tub lung: presenting features and clinical course of 21 patients. Respir Med 2006; 100:610-15.

Henry MT, Inamdar L, O'Riordain D, Schweiger M, Watson JP. Nontuberculous mycobacteria in non.HIV patients:epidemiology, treatment and response. Eur Resp J. 2004;23:741-6.

Iseman MD, Marras TK. The importance of nontuberculous mycobacterial lung disease. Am J Respir Care Med 2008; 178:999-1000.

Jenkins PA, Campbell IA, Banks J, Gelder CM, Prescott RJ et al. Clarithromycin vs ciprofloxacin as adjuncts to rimfapicin and etambutol in treating opportunist mycobacterial lung disease and assessment of Mycobacterium vaccae immunotherapy. Thorax 2008; 63:627-34.

Jeong YJ, Lee KS, Koh WJ, Han J, Kim TS, Kwon OJ. Nontuberculous Mycobacterial Pulmonary Infection in Immunocompetent Patients: Comparison of Thin-Section CT and Histopathologic Findings. Radiology, 2004; 231:880-886.

Kim RD, Greenberg DE, Ehrmantraut ME, Guide SV, Ding L, Shea Y, Brown MR, Chernik M, Stegall WK, Glasgow CG, et al. Pulmonary nontuberculous mycobacterial disease: prospective study of a distinct pre-existing syndrome. Am J Respir Crit Care Med 2008;178:1066-1074.

Kobashi YMT. Comparison of clinical features in patients with pulmonary Mycobacterium avium complex (MAC) disease treated before and after proposal for guidelines. J Infect Chemother 2004;10:25-30.

Leitritz L, Schubert S, Bucherl B, Masch A, Heesemann J et al. Evaluation of BACTEC MGIT 960 and BACTEC 460TB systems for recovery of mycobacteria from clinical specimens of a university hospital with low incidence of tuberculosis. J Clin Microbiol 2001;39:3764-7.

Marras TK, Chedore P, Ying AM, Jamieson F. Isolation of pulmonary non-tuberculous mycobacteria in Ontario, 1997-2003. Thorax 2007; 62:661-666.

Marusic A, Katalinic-Jankovic V, Popovic-Grle S, Jankovic M, Mazuranic I, Puljic I, Sertic Milic H. Mycobacterium xenopi pulmonary disease - epidemiology and clinical features in non-immunocompromised patients. J Infect. 2009; 58(2):108-12.

Martin-Casabona N, Bahrmand AR, Bennedsen J, Thomsen VO, Curcio M et al. Non-tuberculous mycobacteria: patterns of isolation. A multi-country retrospective survey. Int J Tuberc Lung Dis. 2004; 8:1186-93.

Moore EH .Atypical mycobacterial infection in the lung: CT appearance. Radiology 1993; 187(3):777-82.

Patz EF Jr, Swensen SJ, Erasmus J. Pulmonary manifestations of nontuberculous Mycobacterium. Radiol Clin North Am. 1995; 33(4):719-29.

Petrini B. Non-tuberculous mycobacterial infections. Scand J Infect Dis. 2006; 38(4):246-55.

Prince DS, Peterson D.D., Steiner RM, Gottlieb JE, Scott R, Israel HL, Figueroa WG, Fish JE. Infection with Mycobacterium avium complex in patients withouth predisposing conditions. N Engl J Med 1989; 321:863-868.

Reich JM, Johnson RE. Mycobacterium avium complex pulmonary disease presenting as an isolated lingular or middle lobe pattern. The Lady Windermere syndrome. Chest 1992; 101:1605-9.

Runyon E. Typical mycobacteria: their classification. Am. Rev. Respir Dis 1965; 91:288-9

Runyon EH. Anonymous mycobacteria in pulmonary disease. Med Clin North Am 1959; 43:273-90.

Sanchez-Alarcos J, de Miguel-Diez J, Bonilla I, Sicilia J, Alvarez-Sala J. Pulmonary infection due to Mycobacterium szlugai. Respiration 2003; 70:533-6.

Subcommittee of the Joint Tuberculosis Committee of the British Thoracic Society (2000) Management of opportunist mycobacterial infection: Joint Tuberculosis Committee guidelines. 1999; Thorax 55:210–218.

The Research Committee of the British Thoracic Society. First randomised trial of treatments for pulmonary disease caused by. M. avium-intracellulare, M. malmoense and M. xenopi in HIV negative patients: rifampicin, ethambutol and isoniazid versus rifampicin and ethambutol. Thorax 2001;56:167-72.

Thomsen VO, Andersen AB, Miörner H. Incidence and clinical significance of non-tuberculous mycobacteria isolated from clinical specimens during a 2-y nationwide survey. Scand J Infect Dis. 2002; 34(9):648-53.

Thomson RM, Yew WW. When and how to treat pulmonary nontuberculous mycobacterial disease. Respirology. 2009;14:12-26.

Tortoli E, Pecorari M, Fabio G, Messino M, Fabio A. Commercial DNA Probes for Mycobacteria Incorrectly Identify a Number of less Frequently Encounted Species. J Clin Microbiol 2010; 48: 307-310.

van Ingen J, Boeree MJ, de Lange WC, Hoefsloot W, Bendien SA, Magis-Escurra C, Dekhuijzen R, van Soolingen D. Mycobacterium xenopi clinical relevance and determinants, the Netherlands. Emerg Infect Dis. 2008; 14(3):385-9.

Varadi RG, Marras TK. ulmonary Mycobacterium xenopi infection in non-HIV- infected patients: a systematic review. Int J Tuberc Lung Dis. 2009; 13(10):1210-8.

# 5

# Pulmonary Infections

Nalini Gupta and Arvind Rajwanshi
*Department of Cytology and Gynaecological Pathology, Postgraduate Institute of Medical Education and Research, Chandigarh India*

## 1. Introduction

Infections in the respiratory tract are very common but majority involve the upper respiratory system. Pneumonia is usually caused by inhalation of infecting organisms or the same may reach the lung via bloodstream. Pulmonary pathogens can cause tissue damage by a direct invasive cytolytic process or by releasing toxins (endotoxins and/or exotoxins). Acute inflammation may lead to complete resolution, destructive pneumonia with abscess formation, healing by fibrosis or chronic inflammation. Various infective agents causing pneumonia include viruses, bacteria, Mycobacteria, fungi, Chlamydiae, Mycoplasmas or parasites.

The diagnosis of various pulmonary infections is initially based on radiological evaluation depending upon chest X-ray, CT scan or MRI (magnetic resonance imaging). Cytological techniques used for detection of pulmonary infections include sputum examination, bronchial washing & brushing, bronchoalveolar lavage, transbronchial/ transthoracic fine needle aspiration (FNA) and EUS (endoscopic ultrasonography) guided FNA. Transbronchial lung biopsies are performed for histopathological detection of various infections and for histological evidence of invasion. Tissue can be obtained by these techniques for culture or other molecular diagnostic techniques such as polymerase chain reaction (PCR). Special stain most commonly used for bacteria is Gram's stain and for fungi are Gomori's methenamine silver (GMS), Gridley's fungus (GF), and periodic acid-Schiff (PAS) stains.

## 2. Viral infection

Various viruses implicated in viral pneumonia include *influenza, parainflenza, adenovirus, coxsackie, echovirus, varicella, vaccinia* and *measles*. Most viral pneumonias are mild, but may be more severe or may be complicated by secondary bacterial infection.[1] Microscopically, there may be a diffuse pan-lobular pneumonia characterised by extensive proteinaceous exudative material in alveoli with alveolar wall thickening and infiltration by lymphocytes. Hyaline membranes can be formed lining the alveoli. There may be focal interstitial pneumonia. Cytomegalovirus infection is characterised by cytomegaly with a large eosinophilic intranuclear inclusion surrounded by a pale halo giving an owl's eye appearance.[2] Herpes Simplex Virus (HSV) pneumonia is characterized by intranuclear inclusions with nucleomegaly and basophilic ground-glass alterations in the nucleoplasm.[3]

## 3. Bacterial infection

The bacterial infection in lung usually starts with the introduction of organisms into the airways. The routes by which bacteria can reach air spaces are inhalation of an aerosol, aspiration of respiratory or gastrointestinal secretions, or bacteraemic spread.[4,5] The common bacilli include *Streptococcus pneumoniae, Haemophilus influenzae,* anaerobic bacteria, *Staphylococcus aureus,* enteric gram-negative bacilli, *Pseudomonas* spp., *Acinetobacter* spp., *Mycobacterium tuberculosis and Legionelia* spp.

This usually leads to acute inflammation characterized by sheets of polymorphonuclear neutrophils (figure 1), histiocytes, nuclear debris and necrosis which results in tissue destruction in the form of extensive necrotizing pneumonia with lung abscesses. Long-standing infection can lead to nonspecific chronic inflammation predominated by lymphocytes and histiocytes. Chronic pneumonia is most commonly caused by Mycobacteria and fungi. *Actinomyces* spp., *Nocardia* spp., and *Pseudomonas pseudomallei can* produce such infections. Legionnaire's disease is an acute respiratory infection caused by *Legionella pneumophila,* which stains best in tissue with a silver-based Dieterle stain rather than a Gram stain. Organising pneumonia is characterised by intra-alveolar proliferation of fibroblasts producing nodular structures called Masson bodies.

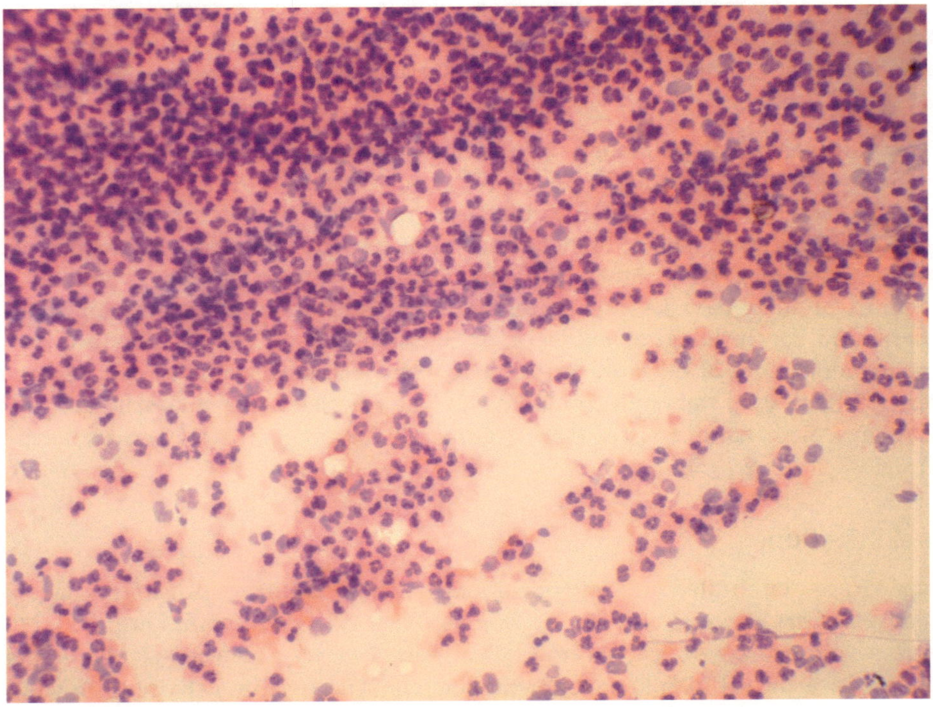

Fig. 1. Sheets of acute inflammatory cells in suppurative inflammation (MGG, 10X)

### 3.1 Granulomatous inflammation

**Granulomatous Inflammation** is characterized by collection of epithelioid histiocytes and multinucleated giant cells. These epithelioid cells may have an elongated cone like shapes or may look like tiny carrots in sputum. These need to be differentiated from bronchial epithelial cells as these are elongated columnar cells which can mimic epithelioid cells.[6]

**Tuberculosis (TB)**

TB can involve various organs but the most common organ involved is lung. TB is more common in the Third World/ developing countries and is much rarer in Western Europe and North America. Primary pulmonary TB usually affects the lower lobes of lung or the anterior segment of an upper lobe, known as the Ghon focus. Microscopically, there are caseating epithelioid granulomas with Langhan's type of multinucleated giant cells and lymphocytes (figure 2 & 3).[7] In tuberculosis, epithelioid histiocytes may be found in about 25% to 50% of sputum specimens.[8] Mycobacteria are identified as elongated beaded acid-fast bacilli (AFB) by Ziehl-Neelsen staining. Auramine-rhodamine stain is another fluorescent dye used to identify these bacilli. Microbiological culture is done using Lowenstein-Jensen medium or Bactec culture. The necrotizing granulomas may be seen in fungal infections or Wegener's granulomatosis. Sarcoidosis is characterised by non-caseating epithelioid granulomas. Secondary pulmonary TB is usually due to re-infection and the lesion is almost always found in the subapical region of an upper lobe. Miliary TB results from seeding of the bacilli via the bloodstream.

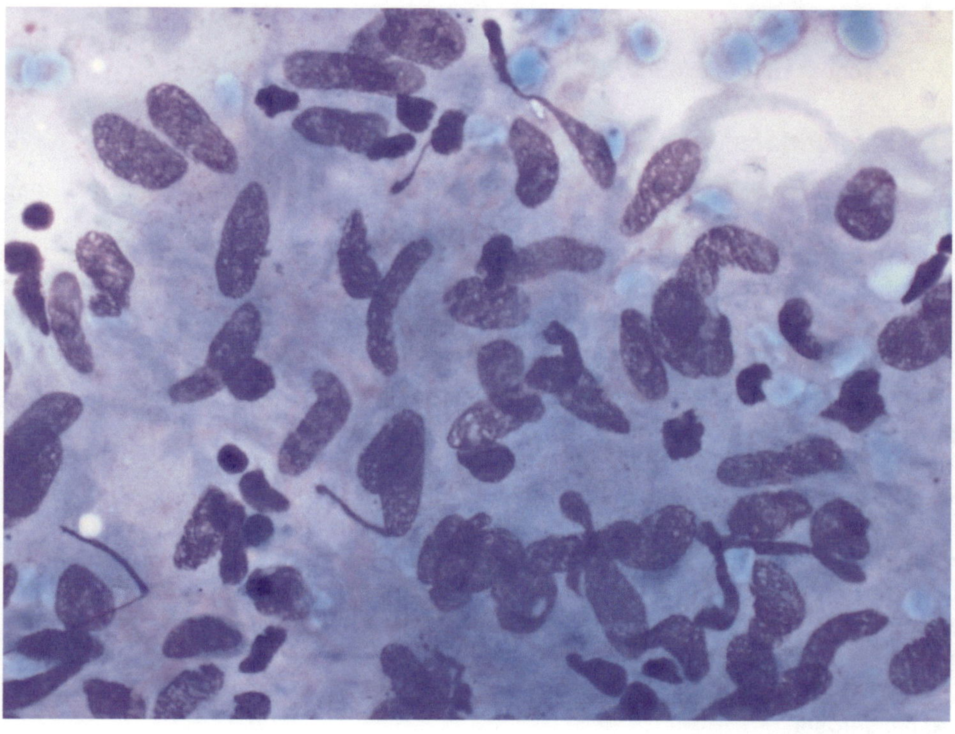

Fig. 2. Epithelioid cell collection and lymphocytes forming a granuloma (MGG, 40X)

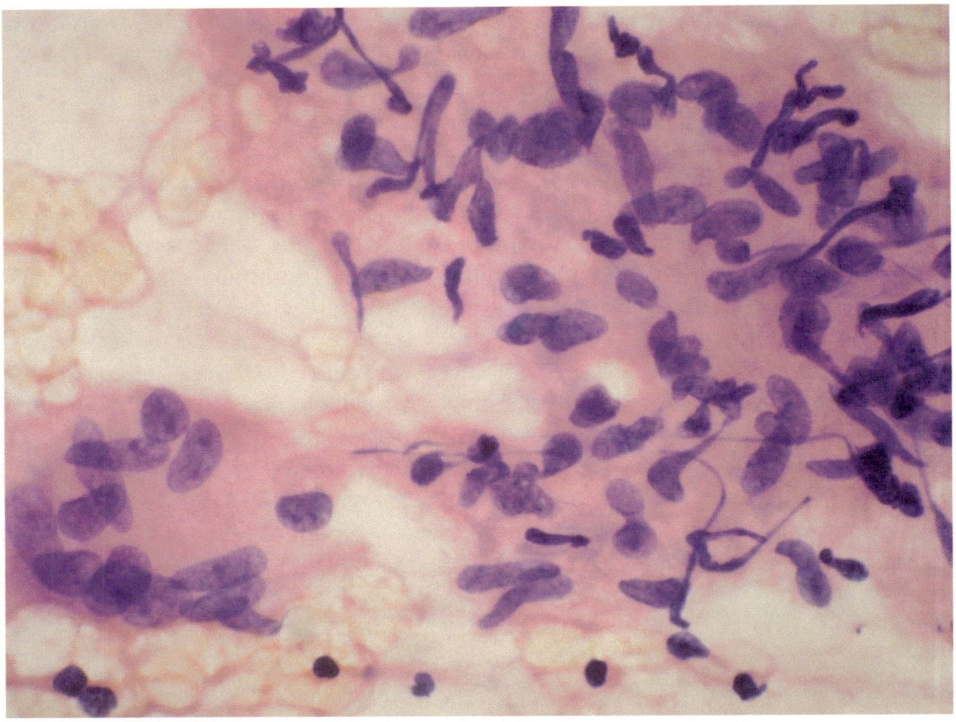

Fig. 3. Epithelioid cell collections in a case of tuberculosis (H&E, 40X)

## 4. Fungal infections

Fungi are eukaryotic, unicellular to multicellular, or filamentous organisms, that are ubiquitous in nature. The incidence of fungal infections is increased over the last two decades mostly because of increase in immunocompromised patients.[9] The incidence of fungal infections in solid organ transplant recipients is between 5-42% and in bone marrow transplant recipients, the incidence ranges between 15-25% with *Aspergillus, Cryptococcus* and *Candida* being the most common fungal infections in these patients.[10,11]

Fungi can elicit various types of tissue reactions such as acute inflammatory, necrosis, granulomatous inflammation. The ability to cause disease depends upon the virulence and the dose of the fungus, the route of infection, immunological status of the host and the organ affected. Lung is one of the most commonly affected organs by opportunistic fungal infections. Majority of the lung infections begin by inhalation of aerosolized fungi from the surrounding environment.[12] The fungi causing invasive pulmonary infection can be primary and opportunistic type of fungi. The primary fungal infection occurs in healthy immunocompetent individuals and the opportunistic fungal infections are common in immunocompromised hosts.

### 4.1 Aspergillosis

The range of disease caused by fungi of the genus *Aspergillus* include- allergic bronchopulmonary disease, colonization of lung cavities/ intracavitory aspergilloma, chronic necrotizing bronchial aspergillosis (CNBA), chronic necrotizing pulmonary aspergillosis (CNPA) in mildly immunocompromised individuals and fulminant invasive pulmonary aspergillosis (IPA) with systemic involvement in severely immunocompromised patients.[13,14] *A fumigatus* (most common), *A flavus, A niger*, and other *Aspergillus* spp. are the common species causing pulmonary infections.[15]

**Allergic pulmonary reactions** occur due to hypersensitivity to Aspergillus antigens especially in patients of bronchial asthma. These include allergic bronchopulmonary aspergillosis, chronic eosinophillic pneumonia, eosinophillic bronchiolitis, mucoid impaction of proximal bronchi or bronchocentric granulomatosis.[16,17] On microscopy, there is an excess of eosinophillic infiltration with Charcot-Leyden crystals, mucus hypersecretion and destructive granulomatous inflammation with degenerated fungal hyphae.[16]

**Pulmonary aspergilloma or fungal/ mycotic ball** is a compact mass of fungal hyphae colonizing pre-existing pulmonary cavity.[14] The cavity may be due to tuberculosis, sarcoidosis, necrotic pulmonary malignancy, bronchiectasis or a bronchial cyst.[18] Majority of the patients develop hemoptysis and the diagnosis is suspected after radiologic detection of thick walled pulmonary cavity with intracavitory mass and a positive serum precipitin reaction to *Aspergillus* antigen.[19]

**Chronic necrotizing bronchial aspergillosis (CNBA)** includes superficial extensive infection of mucosal surface of bronchi resulting in mucosal erosion and ulceration with formation of pseudo-membranes. The patients usually present with wheezing, non-productive cough and dyspnea.

**Chronic necrotizing pulmonary aspergillosis (CNPA)** is a progressive and destructive lesion in mildly immunocompromised individuals with non-cavitary structural lung disease such as sarcoidosis, chronic pulmonary obstructive disease, postradiation fibrosis, diabetes mellitus, tuberculosis, and pneumoconiosis etc. Majority of these patients have history of treatment with low-dose corticosteroids.[20] Treatment includes surgical resection or antifungal therapy with drainage of the pulmonary cavity.

**Invasive pulmonary aspergillosis (IPA)** is a fulminant infection in severely immunocompromised hosts. Vascular invasion is the hallmark of this condition and leads to thrombotic occlusion of arteries and veins. Chest X-ray shows patchy, multifocal or diffuse areas of consolidation, or wedge shaped pleura based infarct like infiltrates or miliary nodules.[21] On microscopy, the nodular infarcts are composed of central ischemic necrosis, surrounded by fibrinous exudates and a peripheral zone of hemorrhage forming a target lesion. Fungal hyphae invade by radial growth and extend from a central occluded vessel. Occlusion of larger vessels lead to formation of wedge shaped pleura-based haemorrhagic infarcts. Disseminated systemic infection occurs in a quarter of patients with IPA involving gastrointestinal tract, central nervous system, kidneys, heart, liver, spleen and thyroid gland.[22]

On microscopic examination, the hyphae of the *Aspergillus* spp. are uniform, narrow (3-6μm in width), septate with regular, progressive and dichotomous branching usually at acute angles (45° angle) from the parent hyphae (figure 4). Conidiophores (fruiting bodies) are seen in lesions exposed to air such as pulmonary/ bronchial lesions. The fungal infection may result in necrotizing or granulomatous inflammation (figure 5) and sometimes is associated with Splendore- Hoeppli phenomenon.

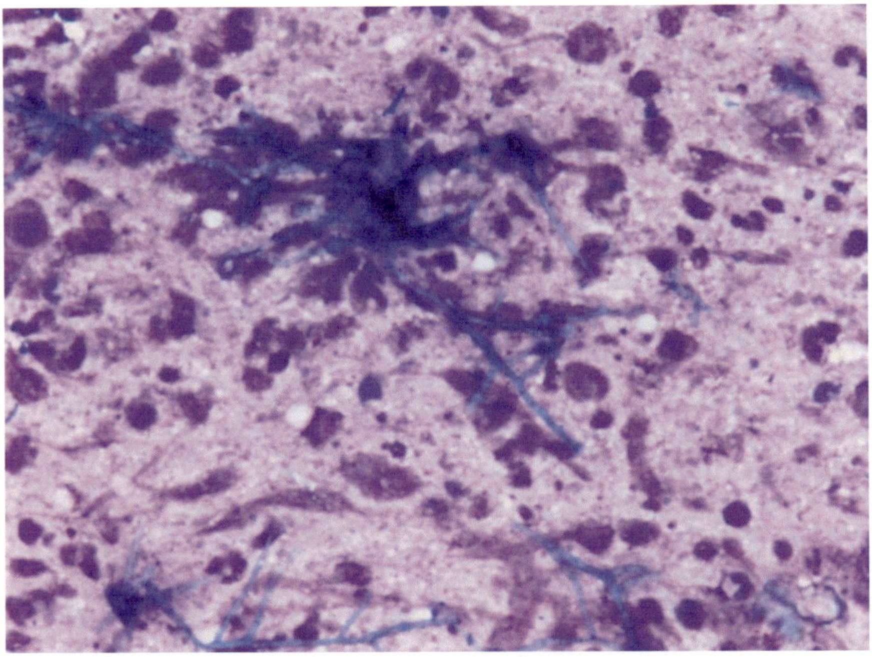

Fig. 4. A long septate hyphae with parallel cell walls of aspergillus in a necrotic background (MGG, 40X)

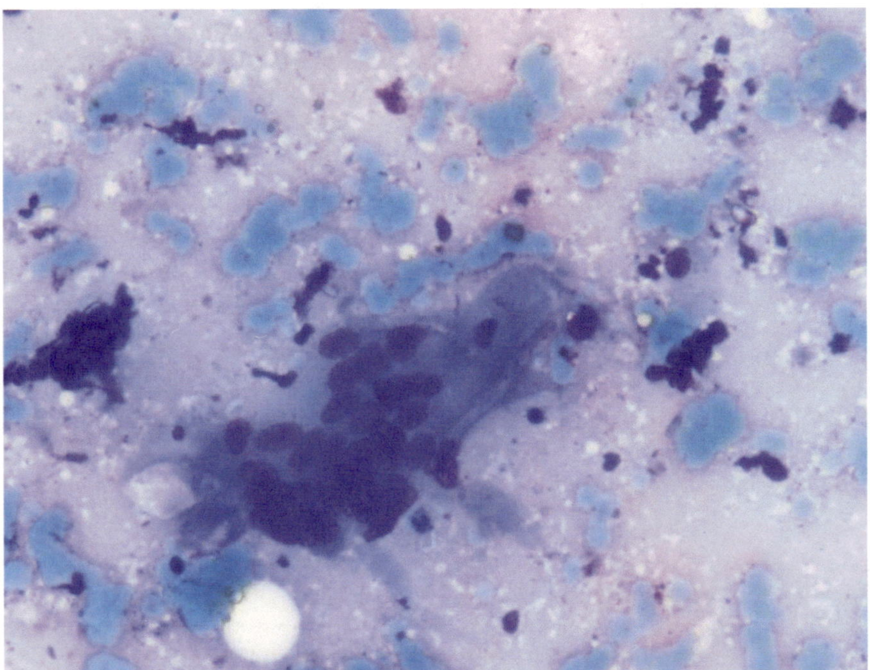

Fig. 5. Occasional hyphae of aspergillus in the multinucleated giant cell (MGG, 40X)

**Differential diagnosis-** The main differential diagnosis of *Aspergillus* includes *zygomycetes, Pseudoallescheria boydii,* the *Fusarium* spp. and occasionally *Candida* spp.

**Treatment-** Amphotericin B is the drug of choice followed by Itraconazole or Voriconazole. Localized infections or aspergilloma may be subjected to surgical excision.

### 4.2 Mucormycosis (Zygomycosis)

Mucormycosis is an opportunistic infection that occurs in immunocompromised hosts especially in patients with acute leukemia or lymphoma, patients treated with corticosteroids, cytotoxic drugs or antibiotic therapy or patients with relapse of an underlying pulmonary disease.[23,24] The agents of mucormycosis include species within the genera *Rhizopus, Absidia, Mucor, Rhizomucor, Saksenaea, Cunninghamella, Mortierella, Syncephalastrum,* and *Apophysomyces.* These fungi are widely distributed and the infection is acquired by exposure to their sporangiospores. The patients usually present with fever and progressive pulmonary infiltrates. Chest X-ray usually shows patchy infiltrates, and single or multiple foci of consolidation.[25]

On microscopic examination, the hyphae of mucormycosis are broad (6-25μm or more wide), delicate thin-walled, aseptate, pleomorphic with irregular non-parallel contours. The branching is often irregular arising at right angles to the parent hyphae. The hyphae are often wrinkled and folded upon themselves. The fungal infection is characterized by coagulative necrosis, neutrophilic infiltration and rarely granulomatous reaction. Angioinvasion leads to disseminated infection and ischemic necrotic lesions and infarcts. Amphotericin B is the drug of choice.

### 4.3 Cryptococcosis

Cryptococcosis starts as lung infection acquired by inhalation of the soil-inhabiting yeast, *Crytococcus neoformans.*[26,27] The fungus is ubiquitous and is especially abundant in aviun, particularly pigeon excreta.[28,29] Although the disease occurs in apparently healthy individuals, it is more often seen as an opportunistic infection especially in patients with haematologic malignancies, AIDS or patients with defective cellular immunity.[30]

The pulmonary lesions include diffuse miliary lesions or patchy consolidation of mucoid nature, which is appreciable in freshly sectioned lungs. On microscopy, cryptococci are of variable size (5-15 μm in diameter) present both intra as well as extracellularly. These are ovoid, thin-walled, encapsulated organisms surrounded by a wide, clear capsule and have narrow-based budding (figure 6). This infection may be accompanied by little or no inflammation, a mixed inflammatory response or a granulomatous reaction. The capsule of these organisms is highlighted on PAS-AB (PAS- Alcain blue) or mucicarmine stains.[31] Autofluorescence microscopy in Papanicolaou-stained smears gives auto fluorescence, which helps in rapid diagnosis of cryptococosis.[32] Cryptococci should be differentiated from Blastomycosis, *Histoplasma capsulatum*, and *Coccidiodes immitis.* The combination of amphotericin B and 5-fluorocytosine is used for progressive pulmonary cryptococcosis.

### 4.4 Histoplasmosis

Histoplasmosis is a pulmonary disease caused by inhalation of airborne infectious conidia of the dimorphic fungus, *Histoplasma capsulatum* var. *capsulatum.*[33] Avian habitat like chicken

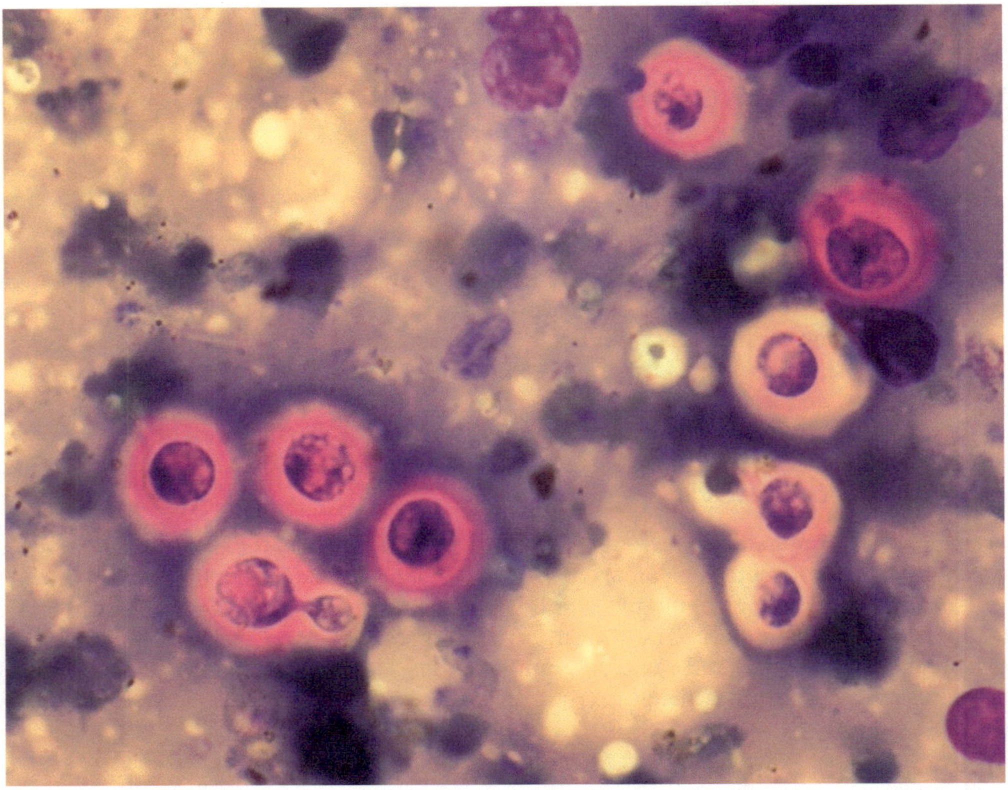

Fig. 6. Extra cellular organisms of Cryptococcus; about 5-15 μm in diameter with budding (MGG, 100X)

coops, blackbird roosts, and caves, favor growth and multiplication of the fungus in soil rich in faecal matter. The clinical presentation depends upon the extent of exposure, presence of underlying pulmonary disease and the host immune status. Majority of the infections are asymptomatic. Symptomatic infection occurs in about 10-25% cases and these can be acute pulmonary disease, disseminated disease, chronic pulmonary disease and fibrosing mediastinitis. The confirmation of the recent or past infection is done by a positive reaction to the cutaneous test antigen histoplasmin.

**Acute pulmonary disease**

The patients may be asymptomatic or develop influenza-like symptoms after an incubation period of about 15 days. Pathologically, the lesion shows bronchopneumonia with neutrophilic infiltration, along with macrophages, lymphocytes, and plasma cells. Granulomatous reaction with multinucleated giant cells occurs after two weeks followed by caseous necrosis.[34]

**Disseminated disease**

Disseminated Histoplasmosis occurs in patients with defective cell mediated immunity and it leads to spread to infection to multiple organs. The patients present with fever with chills, productive cough, hemoptysis, dyspnea, weight loss, headache, drowsiness, diarrhea, generalized lymphadenopathy, hepatosplenomegaly, purpura, and intestinal ulcerations. Chest X-ray usually reveals diffuse pulmonary interstitial infiltrates.[35] The fungi may be associated with granulomatous reaction and the necrotic lesions may calcify.

**Chronic pulmonary Histoplasmosis**

Radiologically, the lesions can be infiltrative, cavitary, fibrosis with emphysema, and the residual solitary nodule or histoplasmoma (coin lesion).[35] Other findings can be military calcification, pleural thickening, and enlarged hilar nodes.

**Fibrosing mediastinitis**

It is a benign condition comprising of fibrosis/ collagenization in mediastinum.[36] The patients present with cough, dyspnea, hemoptysis, and pleurisy. Extensive fibrosis may lead to entrapment of heart or great vessels rarely.

The organisms are yeast like spherical or oval, uniform, 2- 4μm in diameter organisms, which reproduce by single budding (figure 7).[37] The basophilic cytoplasm of the organism is retracted from rigid, thin, poorly stained cell wall, creating a halo/ clear space. The organisms are seen mainly within the macrophages. This may be associated with intense granulomatous reaction with caseation necrosis or calcification, which can mimic tuberculosis. The cell wall intensely stains with special stains especially Gomori methenamine silver stain. Gridley, PAS and Haematoxylin & Eosin stains do not reliably demonstrate these organisms.

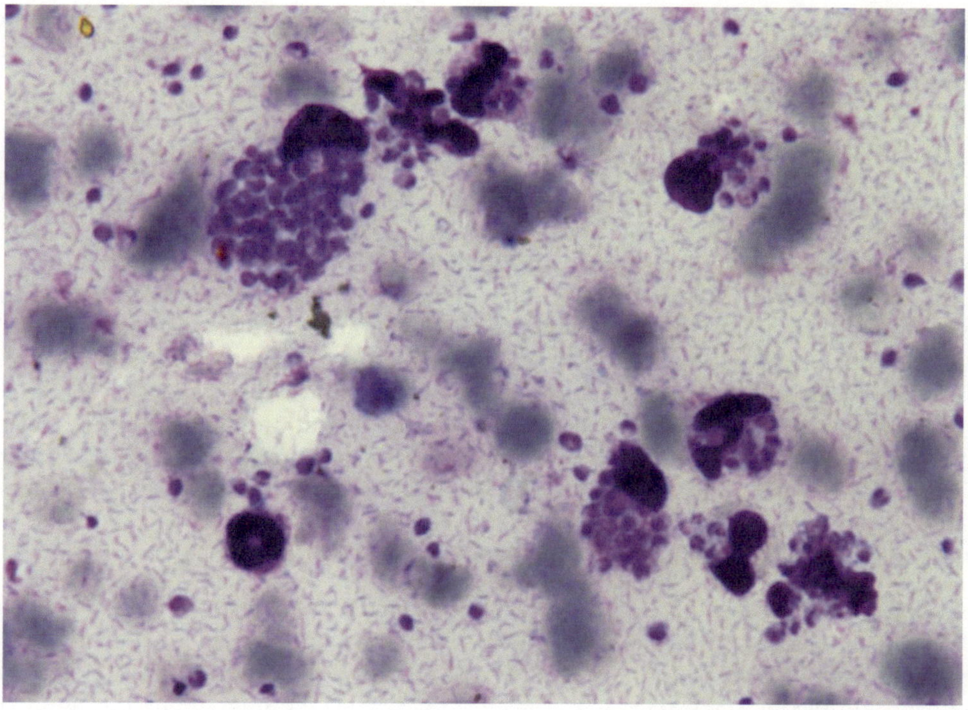

Fig. 7. Extracellular as well as intracellular round to oval, 2-4μm in size, budding yeasts of Histoplasma (MGG, 100X)

**Differential diagnosis-** The differential diagnosis of *Histoplasma capsulatum* includes *Cryptococcus neoformans, Candida glabrata, Coccidiodes immitis, Blastomycosis dermatitidis* and *Leishmania amastigotes.*[37]

## 4.5 Blastomycosis

Blastomycosis is a systemic infection caused by the dimorphic fungus, *Blastomyces dermatitidis.* The infection is acquired by inhalation of airborne conidia of the mycelial form forming a pulmonary focus of infection. The pulmonary involvement can be acute or chronic. Acute pulmonary blastomycosis is usually a self-limited illness and the patient may remain asymptomatic or have non-specific symptoms varying from mild influenza-like symptoms to pneumonia. Chest X-ray shows patchy areas of consolidation with involvement of posterior segments of lower lobes of lungs in majority of the cases. The patients with chronic blastomycosis present with chronic respiratory symptoms such as chronic cough and chest pain persisting for weeks or months.[38] Chest X-ray show linear lung infiltrates, mediastinal lymphadenopathy and pulmonary nodules with cavitation mimicking tuberculosis.[39] Multiple organ involvement occurs involving skin, bone and genitourinary tract.

The infection is acquired by inhalation of conidia from woody plant matter. The mold form is transformed into the yeast form in distal airways. In smears or tissue sections, the yeast is seen intra as well as extracellularly in macrophages and polymorphs. The organism may elicit acute abscess like reaction with neutrophilic infiltration to granulomatous reaction with epithelioid granulomas and multinucleated giant cells. The organisms are round to oval, 8-15µm in diameter with thick refractile double contoured walls and single broad based budding. The differential diagnosis includes *H. capsulatum, Cryptococcus* and *Coccidioides immitis.*

## 4.6 Coccidioidomycosis

It is caused by the dimorphic fungus, *Coccidioides immitis.* It is endemic in the southwest United States[40] and north and central Mexico. Pulmonary infection is acquired by inhalation of airborne arthroconidia. The patients may remain asymptomatic or develop influenza-like illness, which is self-limiting. Chronic pneumonia, destructive fibro-cavitary disease or disseminated infection occurs in minority of the patients. Pulmonary lesions can be pneumonic, cavitary, nodulo-caesous and bronchiectatic.[41] Pulmonary lesions are usually associated with acute suppurative or granulomatous inflammation. The organisms are thin-walled, mature spherules, 30-200µm in diameter (figure 8). Rupture of the spherules releases endospores into the surrounding tissue. The differential diagnosis includes sporangia of *Rhinosporidium seeberi,* budding yeast of *Blastomyces dermatitidis* or *Histoplasma capsulatum.*

## 4.7 Paracoccidioidomycosis (South American blastomycosis)

It is a chronic progressive lung infection caused by *Paracoccidioides brasiliensis* and is endemic in South America. Pulmonary infection may be acute progressive with acute suppurative pneumonia or chronic progressive infection with granulomatous inflammation. The organisms are pleomorphic yeast like, 5-60µm in diameter, reproducing by budding. Yeast cells with fractured walls called mosaic cells are seen in chronic pulmonary lesions. The characteristic multiple budding cells give the appearance of a ship's steering wheel. The

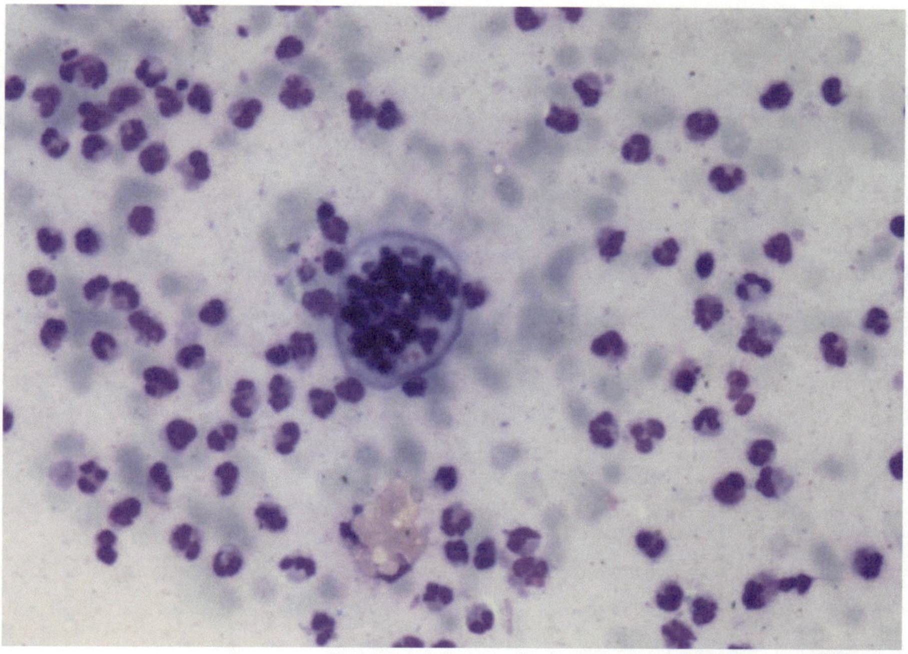

Fig. 8. Thin- walled (30-200μm in diameter) mature spherule of coccidiomycosis (MGG x20X)

blastoconidia produced by these cells can have an oval, tubular appearance or tear-drop blastoconidia attached to the parent cell by narrow necks. This needs to be differentiated from *Histoplasma capsulatum.*

### 4.8 Candidiasis

Candidiasis comprises of superficial, mucocutaneous, or systemic fungal infection caused by yeast like fungi of the genus Candida. *Candida albicans* is the most common type. Pulmonary involvement can be a) endobronchial/ primary pulmonary candidiasis acquired by aspiration of Candida spp. from oral cavity or upper respiratory tract, b) hematogenous pulmonary candidiasis and c) embolic pulmonary candidiasis in children with indwelling venous catheters.[42,43] The lesions contain yeast forms and mycelial forms of Candida. The yeast-like cells are round to oval, 2-6μm in diameter, and have budding. The mycelia forms have both pseudohyphae and true septate branched hyphae. Pseudohyphae have periodic constrictions at the point where budding yeast cells are joined end to end. The inflammatory response to candida may vary from minimal inflammation to acute suppuration to granulomatous inflammation in chronic infections. The differential diagnosis includes *B. dermatitidis,* C. *neoformans, H. capsulatum,* and S. *schenckii,* the tissue forms of these consist of yeast forms.

### 4.9 *Pneumocystis jeroveci*

This is commonly seen in AIDS patients.[44] Microscopically, the alveoli are usually filled with frothy, eosinophilic, PAS-positive coagulum in which the shadows of the non-staining cysts are seen. Grocott's Methenamine Silver (GMS) stain is used and the cell wall of the cyst stains black, often with a central dark dot. The cysts are 4 to 6 μm in diameter and spherical or cup/ sickle-shaped. Trophozoites may be up to 8 per cyst, are about 0.5 to 1.0μm in diameter and stain in Romanowsky (tiny purple dots). The diagnosis may be made on sputum or bronchoalveolar lavage fluid by demonstrating the cysts.

## 5. Bacterial infections that resemble fungal infections

### 5.1 Nocardiosis

Nocardiosis is a localized or disseminated infection caused by aerobic, filamentous, branching gram-positive bacteria.[45] It is an uncommon infection in immunocompetent hosts. Pulmonary lesions may be large cavitating abscesses or diffuse fibrino-suppurative pneumonia. The smears or tissue sections show thin (about 1μm wide), filamentous, beaded bacilli branching at approximately right angles (figure 9).[46] These are usually obscured by an intense acute necrotizing inflammation as they remain unstained on May-Grünwald Geimsa (MGG) stain, Haematoxylin or Eosin (H&E) or PAS stains. The special stain used for its confirmation is a modified Ziehl- Neelsen stain using a weak decolorizing agent.[47] The main differential diagnosis is *Mycobacterium tuberculosis* and *Actinomycosis* (figure 10).

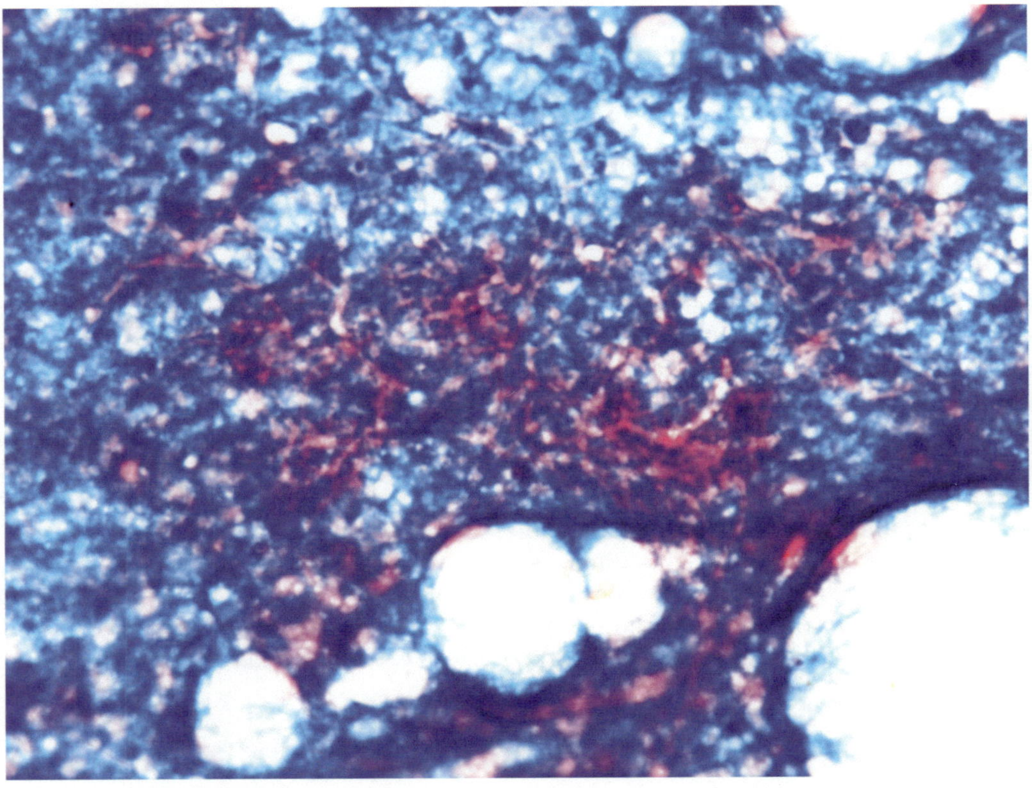

Fig. 9. Multiple long thin filamentous structures (Nocardia) in an inflammatory background (Modified Ziehl- Neelsen stain, 100X).

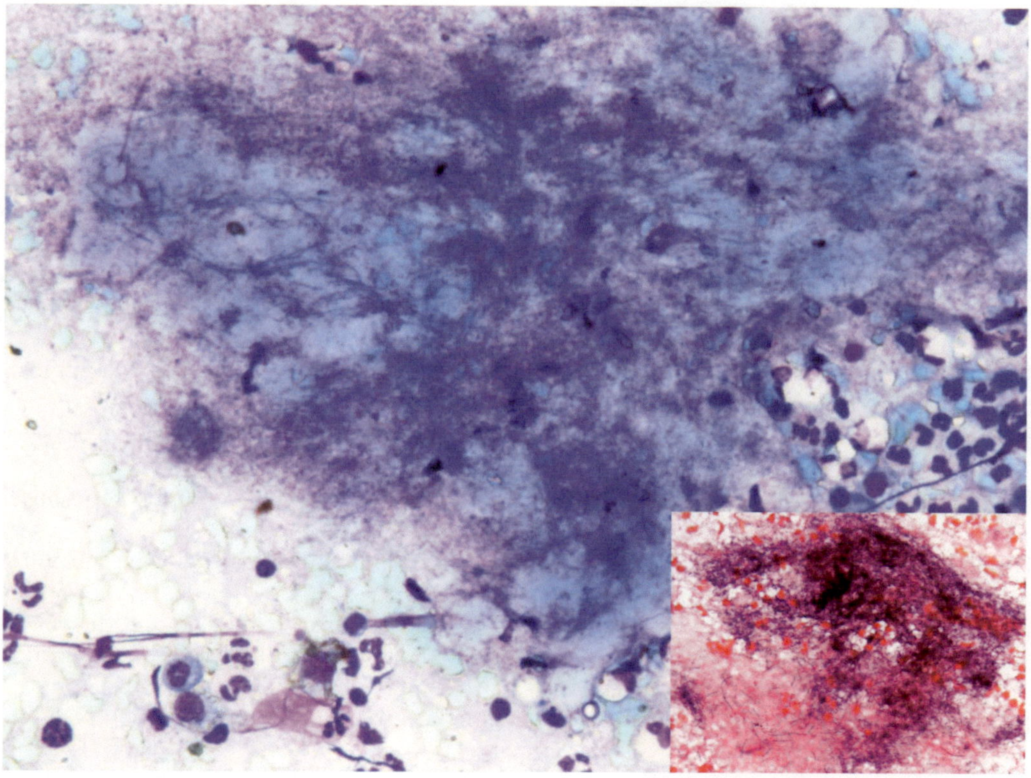

Fig. 10. Filamentous bacilli positive on Gram's stain of Actinomycosis (MGG x40X; Inset-Gram stain- 40X).

### 5.2 Botryomycosis (Bacterial pseudomycosis)

It is a chronic, localized infection of the skin and subcutaneous tissue or various organs including lung and brain.[48] It is caused by non-filamentous bacilli that form granules which include *Pseudomonas aeruginosa, Staphylococcus aureus, Escherichia coli* or *Streptococci.* Pulmonary lesions lead to acute suppurative abscesses with multiple granules which are bordered by eosinophillic, club-like Splendore-Hoeppli material. The differential diagnosis includes nocardiosis and actinomycosis.

## 6. Primary atypical pneumonia

*Mycoplasma pneumoniae* & Chlamydiae are the important causes of primary atypical pneumonia. Mycoplasma can be stained by Giemsa but not by Gram's stain and the diagnosis is usually confirmed serologically. Microscopically, a prominent interstitial infiltrate of lymphocytes, histiocytes and plasma cells is seen with interstitial oedema.

## 7. References

[1] Ruuskanen O, Lahti E, Jennings LC, Murdoch DR. Viral pneumonia. Lancet 2011;377:1264-75.

[2] Miles PR, Baughman RP, Linnemann CC. Cytomegalovirus in the bronchoalveolar lavage fluid of patients with AIDS. Chest. 1990; 97:1072-6.
[3] Chiche L, Forel JM, Papazian L. The role of viruses in nosocomial pneumonia. Curr Opin Infect Dis. 2011;24:152-6.
[4] Griñan NP, Lucena FM, Romero JV, et al. Yield of percutaneous needle lung aspiration in lung abscess. Chest. 1990; 97:69-74.
[5] Palmer DL, Davidson M, Lusk R. Needle aspiration of the lung in complex pneumonias. Chest. 1980; 78:16-21.
[6] Rajwanshi A, Gupta N. Role of FNAC in lung lesions. In: Textbook of Pulmonary & Critical Care Medicine. Jindal SK (editor); Jaypee Brothers Medical Publishers (P) Ltd, New Delhi, 2011; p399-416.
[7] Rajwanshi A, Bhambhani S, Das DK. Fine needle aspiration cytology of tuberculosis. Diagn Cytopathol. 1987; 3:13-6.
[8] Tani EM, Schmitt FC, Oliveira ML et al. Pulmonary cytology in tuberculosis. Acta Cytol. 1987; 31:460-3.
[9] Zupanic-Krmek D, Nemet D. Systemic fungal infections in immunocompromised patients. Acta Med Croatica 2004;58:251-261.
[10] Paya CV. Fungal infections in solid-organ transplantation- Review. Clin Infect Dis 1993;16:677-688.
[11] Visco li C, Castagnola E. Emerging fungal pathogens, drug resistance and the role of lipid formulations of amphotericin B in the treatment of fungal infections in cancer patients: a review. Int J Infect Dis 1999;3:109-118.
[12] Newhouse M, Sanchis J, Bienenstock 1. Lung defense mechanisms (part I). N Engl J Med 1976;295:990-998.
[13] Tsuji S, Ogawa K. Chronic pulmonary aspergillosis. Nihon Rinsho. 2011;69:1462-7.
[14] Kousha M, Tadi R, Soubani AO. Pulmonary aspergillosis: a clinical review. Eur Respir Rev. 2011 Sep 1;20:156-74.
[15] Young RC, Jennings A, Bennett JE. Species identification of invasive aspergillosis in man. Am J Clin Pathol 1972;58:554-57.
[16] Katzenstein AL, Liebow AA, Friedman PJ. Bronchocentric granulomatosis, mucoid impaction, and hypersensitivity reactions to the fungi. Am Rev Respir Dis 1975;111:497-537.
[17] Warnock ML, Fennessy J, Rippon J. Chronic eosinophilic pneumonia, a manifestation of allergic aspergillosis. Am J Clin Pathol 1974;62:73-81.
[18] Addrizzo-Harris D, Harkin T, McGinnis G, et al. Pulmonary aspergilloma and AIDS. A comparison of HIV infected and HIV-negative individuals. Chest 1997;111:612-618.
[19] Glimp RA, Bayer AS. Pulmonary aspergilloma: diagnostic and therapeutic considerations. Arch Intern Med 1983;143:303-308.
[20] Palmer LB, Greenberg HE, Schiff MJ. Corticosteroid treatment as a risk factor for invasive aspergillosis in patients with lung disease. Thorax 1991;46:15-20.
[21] Rau WS. *Aspergillus* infections of the lung: radiographical signs. Mycoses 1997;2(suppl 2):25-32.
[22] Morrison VA, Haake RJ, Weisdorf DJ. Non-Candida fungal infections after bone marrow transplantation: risk factors and outcome. Am J Med 1994;96:497-503.
[23] Quan C, Spellberg B. Mucormycosis, pseudallescheriasis, and other uncommon mold infections. Proc Am Thorac Soc. 2010;7:210-5.

[24] Spira A, Brecher S, Karlinsky 1. Pulmonary mucormycosis in the setting of chronic obstructive pulmonary disease. Respiration 2002;69:560-563.
[25] Bartrum RJ, Watnick M, Herman PG. Roentgenographic findings in pulmonary mucormycosis. Am J Roentgenol Radium Ther Nucl Med 1973;117:810-815.
[26] Silva EG, Paula CR, de Assis Baroni F, Gambale W. Voriconazole, combined with Amphotericin B, in the treatment for Pulmonary Cryptococcosis caused by C. neoformans (Serotype A) in mice with Severe Combined Immunodeficiency (SCID). Mycopathologia. 2011 Nov 10. [Epub ahead of print]
[27] Lewis JL, Rabinovich S. The wide spectrum of cryptococcal infections. Am J Med 1972;53:315-322.
[28] Ellis DH, Pfeiffer TJ. The ecology of *Cryptococcus neoformans*. Eur J Epidemiol1992;8:321-325.
[29] Srinivasan R, Gupta N, Shifa R, Malhotra P, Rajwanshi A, Chakrabarti A. Cryptococcal lymphadenitis diagnosed by fine needle aspiration cytology: a report of 15 cases. Acta Cytol 2010; 54: 1-4.
[30] Clark RA, Greer D, Atkinson W, et al. Spectrum of *Cryptococcus neoformans* infection in 68 patients infected with human immunodeficiency virus. Rev Infect Dis 1990;12:768-777.
[31] Garbyal RS, Basu D, Roy S, Kumar P. Cryptococcal lymphadenitis: report of a case with fine needle aspiration cytology. Acta Cytol 2005; 49: 58-60.
[32] Wright CA, Leiman G, Benatar B. Fine needle aspiration of Cryptococcal lymphadenitis: Further observation using autofluorescence. Acta Cytol 2000; 44: 281-282.
[33] Domer JE, Moser SA. Histoplasmosis- a review. Rev Med Vet Mycol 1980;15:159-83.
[34] Goodwin RA Jr, Loyd JE, Des Prez RM. Histoplasmosis in normal hosts. Medicine (Baltimore) 1981;60:231-266.
[35] Connell JW, Muhm JR. Radiographic manifestations of pulmonary histoplasmosis: a 10-year review. Radiology 1976;121 :281-285.
[36] Peikert T, Colby TV, Midthun DE, Pairolero PC, Edell ES, Schroeder DR, Specks U. Fibrosing mediastinitis: clinical presentation, therapeutic outcomes, and adaptive immune response. Medicine (Baltimore). 2011;90:412-23.
[37] Gupta N, Arora SK, Rajwanshi A, Nijhawan R, Srinivasan R. Histoplasmosis-Cytodiagnosis and review of literature with special emphasis on differential diagnosis on cytomorphology. Cytopathol 2010; 21: 240-44.
[38] Vanek J, Schwarz J, Hakim S. North American blastomycosis. Am J Clin Pathol 1970;54:384-400.
[39] Halvorsen RA, Duncan JD, Merten DJ, et al. Pulmonary blastomycosis: radiologic manifestations. Radiology 1984;150:1-5.
[40] Vikram HR, Dosanjh A, Blair JE. Coccidioidomycosis and lung transplantation. Transplantation. 2011;92:717-21.
[41] Huntington RW Coccidioidomycosis. In: Baker RD, ed. The pathologic anatomy of mycoses: human infection with fungi, actinomycetes, and algae. Berlin: Springer-Verlag, 1971:147-210.
[42] Dubois PJ, Myerowitz RL, Allen CM. Pathoradiologic correlation of pulmonary candidiasis in immunosuppressed patients. Cancer 1977;40:1026-36.

[43] Kassner EG, Kauffman SL, Yoon JJ, Semiglia M, Kozinn PJ, Goldberg PL. Pulmonary candidiasis in infants: clinical, radiologic and pathologic features. AJR 1981;137:707-16.
[44] Chaudhary S, Hughes WT, Feldman S, et al. Percutaneous transthoracic needle aspiration of the lung. Diagnosing Pneumocystis carinii pneumonitis. Am J Dis Child. 1977;131:902-7.
[45] Shivaprakash MR, Rao P, Mandal J, et al. Nocardiosis in a tertiary care hospital in North India and review of patients reported from India. Mycopathologica 2007;163:267–274.
[46] Gupta N, Srinivasan R, Kumar R, Chakrabarti A. Two cases of Nocardiosis diagnosed by fine Needle Aspiration Cytology: Role of Special Stains. Diagn Cytopathol 2010;39:363-4.
[47] Mathur S, Sood R, Aron M, Iyer VK, Verma K. Cytologic diagnosis of pulmonary nocardiosis: A report of 3 cases. Acta Cytol 2005;49:567–570.
[48] Vasishta RK, Gupta N, Kakkar N. Botryomycosis - a series of integumentary or visceral cases from India. Annl Trop Med Parasitol 2004;98:623-9.

6

# Host Immune Responses Against Pulmonary Fungal Pathogens

Karen L. Wozniak[1,2], Michal Olszewski[3,4] and Floyd L. Wormley Jr.[1,2,*]
*[1]Department of Biology, The University of Texas at San Antonio, San Antonio, TX*
*[2]South Texas Center for Emerging Infectious Diseases, The University of Texas at San Antonio, San Antonio, TX*
*[3]Veterans Affairs Ann Arbor Health System, Ann Arbor, MI*
*[4]University of Michigan Medical School, Ann Arbor, MI*
*USA*

## 1. Introduction

The lungs are a gateway for numerous airborne pathogens that are ubiquitous in our environment. Among these potential pathogens are fungi that can be found in the soil, bird excreta, air ducts, and many other places where their contact is unavoidable. Exposure to these fungal pathogens oftentimes goes unnoticed due to the activation of our robust immune systems which sequester and control these microbes before significant damage occurs. Still, there are many situations in which host immunity becomes compromised providing an opportunity for typically innocuous fungal organisms to become established and cause disease or for dormant infections to reawaken. Also, in certain cases disease may be exacerbated due to an over exuberant immune response. In this chapter, we will review the main aspects of innate and adaptive immune responses against pulmonary fungal pathogens. We will also discuss the potential for vaccines to prevent pulmonary fungal infections.

## 2. Introduction to pulmonary fungal infections

Pulmonary fungal infections can be grouped into primary fungal pathogens and opportunistic fungal pathogens. Those organisms that can cause disease in immune competent hosts are considered primary pathogens including *Histoplasma capsulatum, Coccidioides immitis, Paracoccidioides brasilensis, and Blastomyces dermatiditis.* All of the primary pulmonary fungal pathogens are endemic to the United States and/or Central & South America. *Histoplasma* and *Blastomyces* are endemic to the Ohio River & Mississippi River Valleys of the United States and also to certain regions of Central and South America (Klein et al., 1986; Deepe, 2000). *Coccidioides* is prevalent in the desert southwest United States (Fisher et al., 2007), and *Paracoccidioides* is endemic in Central and South America, particularly in Brazil (Franco, 1987; Franco et al., 1989; Brummer et al., 1993). These

* Corresponding Author

infections are acquired by inhalation of fungi from contaminated soil, and severity of disease generally correlates with the amount of exposure to the pathogen.

Examples of organisms that are opportunistic pulmonary fungal pathogens include *Cryptococcus neoformans*, *Aspergillus fumigatus*, *Pneumocystis*, and *Rhizopus*. *C. neoformans* is found ubiquitously in the soil, usually in soil contaminated with pigeon guano (Perfect and Casadevall, 2002). These fungi primarily cause disease in individuals with compromised immune systems. Most cryptococcal infections are asymptomatic, and the organism typically causes disease in immune compromised patients, such as AIDS patients, solid organ transplant patients on immune-suppressive drugs, or patients receiving chemotherapy (Levitz, 1991; Mitchell and Perfect, 1995; Singh et al., 1997; Shoham and Levitz, 2005). *A. fumigatus* is ubiquitously found in the environment, and is normally found in association with decaying wood and plant matter (Deacon et al., 2009). However, *A. fumigatus* can cause severe respiratory infections in cases of massive exposure or immune deficiency, such as neutropenia, due to chemotherapy, AIDS, or bone marrow transplant therapy (Denning, 1996; Almyroudis et al., 2005; Magill et al., 2008). *Pneumocystis* infection is acquired by inhalation of organisms from a yet unknown source (Keely et al., 1995; reviewed in Kelly and Shellito, 2010). Most *Pneumocystis* infections occur in immunosuppressed individuals due to either HIV or chronic obstructive pulmonary disease (Leigh et al., 1993; Nevez et al., 1999; Huang et al., 2003; Calderon et al., 1996; Morris et al., 2004; Norris et al., 2006; Davis et al., 2008; Morris et al., 2008a; Morris et al., 2008b; Kling et al., 2009). Similarly, infection with *Rhizopus* typically occurs in individuals who are immune compromised, such as organ transplant recipients (Kontoyiannis, 2010; Pappas et al., 2010).

## 3. Innate immune responses against pulmonary fungal pathogens

### 3.1 Phagocyte interactions with pulmonary fungal pathogens

Cells of the innate immune system such as dendritic cells (DCs) and macrophages residing in the lungs/airways are the first line of defense against pulmonary fungal pathogens. Although these innate cells cannot completely eliminate many fungal pathogens, they are involved in uptake and degradation of fungi and processing of antigens derived from these pathogens. In contrast, neutrophils which are also phagocytic and can be fungistatic are unable to present antigen. Based on the subset of receptors involved and signaling pathways triggered by these receptors, the innate immune system will trigger different types of early responses and subsequently translate these signals to mount different types of adaptive responses.

*H. capsulatum* can initially be engulfed by macrophages, DCs, and neutrophils (reviewed in (Deepe, 2005)), however, *H. capsulatum* recognition by different receptors results in different fates (Gomez et al., 2008). DCs recognize *H. capsulatum* by VLA-5, by interaction with an unknown receptor, which results in uptake, killing, and antigen presentation (Gildea et al., 2001; Gomez et al., 2008). Human DCs exert their antifungal activity via phagolysosomal fusion. The addition of suramin (which blocks phagolysosomal fusion) inhibits DC fungicidal activity, but inhibition of lysosomal acidification and inhibition of respiratory burst has no effect (Gildea et al., 2005). In contrast to DCs, macrophages recognize the *H. capsulatum* surface molecule heat-shock protein 60 (HSP 60) by LFA-1 (CD11a/CD18), complement receptor 3 (CD11b/CD18), and complement receptor 4 (CD11c/CD18) and this recognition leads to uptake and intracellular replication (Kimberlin et al., 1981; Bullock and Wright, 1987; Long et al., 2003; Gomez et al., 2008; Lin et al., 2010). However, activated macrophages can halt intracellular replication (Wu-Hsieh and Howard, 1984; Wu-Hsieh et al., 1984). *H. capsulatum* can avoid the macrophage lysosomal environment by preventing phagolysosomal fusion (Newman et al., 1997; Strasser et al., 1999) or by alkalinizing the pH of the phagolysosome (Eissenberg and Goldman, 1988; Eissenberg et al., 1988; Eissenberg et al., 1993). Macrophages infected with *H. capsulatum* and activated with GM-CSF decrease available iron and zinc, while infected macrophages without GM-CSF do not. Further, chelation of zinc inhibits yeast replication; therefore zinc deprivation may be used by macrophages in host defense against *H. capsulatum* (Winters et al., 2010). Neutrophil phagocytosis of *H. capsulatum* requires opsonization with either antibody or complement (Brummer et al., 1991; Kurita et al., 1991a; Kurita et al., 1991b; Newman et al., 1993). Neutrophil uptake of *H. capsulatum* is fungistatic, as opposed to macrophages (permissive growth & replication) and DCs (fungicidal) (reviewed in Deepe, 2005). A lack of neutrophils causes a non-lethal infection to become a lethal infection (Zhou et al., 1998).

Immature DCs bind spherules of *Coccidioides* in a time and temperature-dependent manner, and binding is blocked by mannan, suggesting that mannose receptor (MR) is involved in this interaction (Dionne et al., 2006). Spherules of *Coccidioides* stimulate DC functional maturation, evidenced by decreased endocytic capacity and stimulation of allogeneic peripheral blood mononuclear cell activation (Dionne et al., 2006). Further studies showed that a DC-based *Coccidioides* vaccine had adjuvant properties and activated protective immune responses in mice (Awasthi, 2007). Although macrophages can ingest *Coccidioides;* earlier studies suggested that they are not able to kill the arthroconidia (Kashkin et al., 1977; Beaman et al., 1981, 1983; Beaman and Holmberg, 1980b, 1980a). Studies demonstrated that monocytes derived from human peripheral blood were able to kill *Coccidioides* (Ampel and Galgiani, 1991). Neutrophils are the earliest cell type to infiltrate upon pulmonary infection with *Coccidioides* arthroconidia (Savage and Madin, 1968). Phagocytosis by neutrophils is enhanced by the addition of immune serum (Drutz and Huppert, 1983; Wegner et al., 1972; Frey and Drutz, 1986). Uptake of *Coccidioides* arthroconidia by neutrophils induces a respiratory burst (Frey and Drutz, 1986), but less than 20% of the arthroconidia are killed (Frey and Drutz, 1986; Beaman and Holmberg, 1980b; Drutz and Huppert, 1983). The spherule form of *Coccidioides* cannot be phagocytosed by or killed by neutrophils (Frey and Drutz, 1986; Galgiani, 1986), but rupture of the spherule leads to an influx of neutrophils (Frey and Drutz, 1986).

*P. brasiliensis* can be phagocytosed by immature DCs, and uptake is significantly decreased with the addition of mannan, suggesting that MR is the primary receptor for *P. brasiliensis* on DCs (Ferreira et al., 2004). After DC uptake of *P. brasiliensis,* the fungal organisms survive and multiply intracellularly rather than being killed (Ferreira et al., 2004). Following *in vitro* culture of *P. brasiliensis* or the major surface antigen gp43 with DCs, major histocompatibility complex (MHC) II is downregulated as is the production of interleukin (IL)-12 and tumor necrosis factor (TNF)-α (Ferreira et al., 2004). However, *in vivo* studies showed that DC interaction with *P. brasiliensis* results in modification of DC receptor expression, including upregulation of CCR7, CD103, and MHC II and also induces migration of both pulmonary and bone marrow-derived DCs. DCs are also able to activate T helper cell responses in the draining lymph nodes following interaction with *P. brasiliensis* (Silvana dos Santos et al., 2011). Alveolar macrophages adhere to and internalize *Paracoccidioides* using the organism's phospholipase B, which also serves to downregulate macrophage activation (Soares et al., 2010). During pulmonary infection with *P. brasiliensis,* a shift in macrophage activation occurs, which is characterized by an increase in IL-1, TNF-α, and IL-6 (Silva et al., 2011). *P. brasilensis* can proliferate within macrophages, but macrophage activation inhibits its growth (Brummer et al., 1988; Cano et al., 1994). Further, macrophages activated by interferon (IFN)-γ can kill *P. brasiliensis* (Cano et al., 1994; Gonzalez et al., 2000). *In vitro* stimulation of human monocytes and neutrophils with *Paracoccidiodes* yeast showed downregulation of toll-like receptor (TLR)2, TLR4, and dectin-1 on the surface of these cells. In addition, yeast cells induced the production of pro-inflammatory cytokines such as TNF-α (Bonfim et al., 2009). Mice lacking TLR2 had a less severe pulmonary infection than wild-type (WT) mice and had decreased nitric oxide (NO) production. However, despite the differences in infection, both TLR2$^{-/-}$ mice and WT mice had similar rates of survival and similar pulmonary inflammatory responses (Loures et al., 2009). Further, TLR2 deficiency skewed the adaptive response towards a T helper (Th)17 phenotype and caused a decrease in T regulatory cells. Increased neutrophils and eosinophils migrate to the lungs of mice susceptible to *P. brasiliensis*, (Cano et al., 1995), and this influx affects the disease outcome and the adaptive response induced to infection. In susceptible individuals recovered from *Paracoccidiodes*, neutrophils are able to phagocytose the organism, but this leads to degeneration of the neutrophils. These data suggest that susceptible individuals have an inherent neutrophil deficiency (Dias et al., 2008). Further, neutrophils from patients with *P. brasiliensis* have a digestive defect against the fungus (Goihman-Yahr et al., 1980), and also have a killing defect against the fungus (Goihman-Yahr et al., 1985; Goihman-Yahr et al., 1992).

*B. dermatiditis* interaction with DCs causes efficient upregulation of antigen presentation and costimulatory molecules and induces production of IL-12 and TNF-α (Wuthrich et al., 2006). DCs can activate CD8$^+$ T cells in the absence of CD4$^+$ T cells, and the yeast alone is a sufficient inflammatory stimulus that can directly induce maturation of DCs and can induce production of TNF-α, IL-1β, and IL-12 (Wuthrich et al., 2006). Monocyte-derived dendritic cells can associate with yeast in the lung and transport them to the draining lymph nodes, but fail to present antigen to CD4$^+$ T cells, however dermal DCs are capable of antigen presentation (Ersland et al., 2010). During *B. dermatiditis* infection, alveolar macrophages are only modestly able to ingest and kill the yeast form of the organism (Bradsher et al., 1987). Murine macrophages are only able to kill less than 5% of yeast (Brummer and Stevens, 1987; Brummer et al., 1988), and had a 25-30% reduction in respiratory burst compared to the respiratory burst induced by zymosan. The *Blastomyces* adhesion 1 (*BAD1*) molecule on the *Blastomyces* yeast surface is responsible for binding to CD11b/CD18 and CD14 on the macrophage surface and subsequent entry (Klein et al., 1993; Newman et al., 1995). Neutrophils rapidly infiltrate to pulmonary tissues following infection, and are responsible for the formation of pyogranulomatous lesions. Conidia are rapidly phagocytosed by neutrophils, but killing of conidia is inefficient. Similar to macrophages, the neutrophil respiratory burst induced by conidia is only 70% of that induced by zymosan (Drutz and Frey, 1985). In addition, yeasts are even more difficult for the neutrophils to phagocytose & kill than conidia (Drutz and Frey, 1985).

*Pneumocystis* interacts with DCs in vitro by MR, (Kobayashi et al., 2007) but the interaction does not lead to an increase in maturation markers such as MHC II, CD40, CD54, CD80, or CD86. Additionally, this interaction induces the production of IL-4 but not IL-12p40, IL-10, TNF-α, or IL-6 (Kobayashi et al., 2007). However, *Pneumocystis* cell wall β-glucans have the ability to induce costimulatory molecule upregulation on DCs, such as MHC II, CD80, CD86, and CD40. These DCs interacted with β-glucans from *Pneumocystis* via dectin-1, and co-stimulatory molecule expression and Th1-type cytokine secretion by β-glucan stimulated DCs was regulated by Fas-Fas ligand interaction (Carmona et al., 2006). *In vivo* administration of DCs pulsed with *Pneumocystis* induced specific T cell responses and release of IL-4 as well as specific $IgG_1$, $IgG_{2a}$, and $IgG_{2b}$ production (Kobayashi et al., 2007). Alveolar macrophages have been shown to directly kill both *Pneumocystis* trophozoites and cysts (Fleury et al., 1985; reviewed in Kelly and Shellito, 2010). Specifically, alternatively-activated macrophages (aaMac) are important effector cells against *Pneumocystis*, and aaMac is enhanced by IL-33 (Nelson et al., 2011). In addition, *Pneumocystis* infection causes changes in gene expression of alveolar macrophages that included upregulation of genes involved in antigen presentation and antimicrobial peptides, but downregulation of genes involved in phagocytosis and uptake (Cheng et al., 2010). *Pneumocystis* major surface glycoprotein (MSG), which is a heavily glycosylated surface antigen, is recognized by MR on alveolar macrophages (Ezekowitz et al., 1991). *Pneumocystis* infection in $HIV^+$ patients induces shedding of the MR, which results in reduced alveolar macrophage phagocytosis of the microbe (Koziel et al., 1998; Fraser et al., 2000). Neutrophils can also interact with *Pneumocystis*, but the presence of neutrophils is correlated with inflammation and increased severity of disease (reviewed in Kelly and Shellito, 2010).

Inhaled *A. fumigatus* conidia are first encountered by alveolar macrophages and neutrophils (reviewed in Hasenberg et al., 2011). Following uptake of *Aspergillus* by phagocytes, the organism enters the phagosome and killing occurs following phagosomal fusion with lysosomes, (Ibrahim-Granet et al., 2003). In the absence or impairment of phagocytic cells, there are dramatic increases in invasive *Aspergillus* infections (Latge, 1999). β-1,3 glucans of *Aspergillus* swollen conidia and hyphae are recognized by dectin-1 on the surface of alveolar macrophages, monocytes, and neutrophils (Taylor et al., 2002; Taylor et al., 2007). This recognition of *Aspergillus* leads to phagocytosis and the production of cytokines such as TNF-α, IL-6, and IL-18 (Gersuk et al., 2006). In addition, *Aspergillus* can be recognized by TLRs, predominantly TLR2 and TLR4 (Wang et al., 2001; Mambula et al., 2002; Netea et al., 2002; Meier et al., 2003; Netea et al., 2003; Bellocchio et al., 2004; Bochud et al., 2008), but phagocytosis and uptake are not due to recognition by TLR2, TLR4, TLR9, or MyD88 (Bellocchio et al., 2004). More recent data also points to recognition of *Aspergillus* unmethylated DNA by TLR9 (Ramirez-Ortiz et al., 2008; Ramaprakash et al., 2009). Further, TLR9 is actively recruited to the *Aspergillus* phagosome and requires the N-terminal proteolytic cleavage domain for proper intracellular trafficking (Kasperkovitz et al., 2010).

DCs bind and internalize *A. fumigatus* through DC-SIGN, and this binding triggers DC maturation (Serrano-Gomez et al., 2004). Mouse DCs can internalize conidia of *A. fumigatus* using MR and a C-type lectin receptor as well as FcγR (Bozza et al., 2002). Upon exposure of DCs to *A. fumigatus*, DCs upregulate HLA-DR, CD80 and CD86 (Grazziutti et al., 2001; Bozza et al., 2002). Following *A. fumigatus* infection, DCs can release the chemokine CXCL8, which promotes migration of PMNs, can upregulate CCL19, which is important in migration of $CCR7^+$ naïve T cells and mature DCs to lymph nodes, and can release soluble factors that increase CD11b and CD18 on PMNs (Gafa et al., 2007). DC phagocytosis of *A. fumigatus* conidia and hyphae occur by different means and through different receptors; conidia are phagocytosed by coiling phagocytosis and hyphae are phagocytosed by zipper-type phagocytosis (Bozza et al., 2002). *A. fumigatus* killing by DCs is dependent on phagolysosomal fusion and a reduction in pH (Ibrahim-Granet et al., 2003). Plasmacytoid DCs (pDCs) have the ability to spread over *A. fumigatus* hyphae and inhibit their growth

(Ramirez-Ortiz et al., 2011), and antifungal activity does not require direct cell contact. Following interaction of pDCs with *Aspergillus*, pDCs release pro-inflammatory cytokines, such as IFN-α and TNF-α, and these are produced via a TLR9-independent mechanism (Ramirez-Ortiz et al., 2011). During the early stages of *Aspergillus* infection, alternatively activated macrophages are recruited to the lung and are important in host defense (Bhatia et al., 2011). Studies examining the interaction of *Aspergillus* conidia with alveolar macrophages showed that infectivity and inhibition of macrophage killing by the fungus were due to the presence of a siderophore system that allows the fungus to acquire iron (Schrettl et al., 2010). In neutropenic mice, inflammatory DCs are recruited to the lungs during *Aspergillus* infection, and this recruitment is dependent on the absence of neutrophils (Park et al., 2010). This accumulation led to increased TNF-α, CCL2, and CCL20, which resulted in further recruitment of inflammatory DCs. Neutrophils, when incubated with *A. fumigatus* hyphae, form neutrophil extracellular traps (NETs), which are antifungal, but mostly act in a fungistatic manner to limit spread of the hyphae (Bruns et al., 2010; Hasenberg et al., 2011).

*In vitro* studies of DCs with *C. neoformans* have shown that DCs are involved in detection, binding, phagocytosis, processing, antigen presentation, T cell activation, and killing of the organism (Bauman et al., 2000; Bauman et al., 2003; Wozniak et al., 2006; Wozniak and Levitz, 2008). DCs isolated from infected lungs presented cryptococcal mannoprotein (MP) to MP-specific T cells and induced T cell activation ex vivo (Wozniak et al., 2006). Depletion of DCs abrogated the T cell response (Mansour et al., 2006). Furthermore, DC phagocytosis of mannoprotein (MP) in the presence of the appropriate adjuvant induces production of Th1-type cytokines (Dan et al., 2008). Additional studies revealed that the interaction of *C. neoformans* with DCs, but not macrophages, induced the production of IL-12 and IL-23, two cytokines associated with protection against cryptococcosis (Kleinschek et al., 2010). Phagocytosis of encapsulated *C. neoformans* by DCs requires opsonization with either anti-capsular antibody or complement, and the combination of these has an additive effect (Kelly et al., 2005). Also, both murine and human DCs are able to kill *C. neoformans*, by both oxidative and non-oxidative mechanisms (Kelly et al., 2005). Recognition and uptake of acapsular *C. neoformans* strains by DCs requires MR and FcγR II (Syme et al., 2002). TLR2 and TLR4 are not important in uptake of *C. neoformans* or activation of DCs by the fungus (Nakamura et al., 2006). DCs stimulated with DNA from *C. neoformans* release IL-12p40 and express CD40, a costimulatory molecule associated with DC maturation, and thus was tied to recognition by TLR9 (Nakamura et al., 2008). Upon infection with *C. neoformans*, CCR2-deficient mice, which are impaired in trafficking of monocyte-derived DCs, developed a non-protective Th2-type immune response and persistent infection, and had reduced DC recruitment, bronchovascular collagen deposition, and increased IL-4 production (Osterholzer et al., 2008). *C. neoformans* can also be phagocytosed by macrophages (Levitz et al., 1999; Del Poeta, 2004). Macrophage phenotypes are associated with differential immune responses against *C. neoformans*. Protection against infection is associated with the presence of classically-activated macrophages (caMac) (Zhang et al., 2009; Hardison et al., 2010a; Hardison et al., 2010b), while disease progression is associated with the presence of alternatively activated macrophages (aaMac) (Arora et al., 2005; Muller et al., 2007; Arora et al., 2011; Chen et al., 2007; Guerrero et al., 2010). Also, macrophages can serve as a site of replication of *C. neoformans* (Tucker and Casadevall, 2002). Intracellular replication rates within macrophages correlated to virulence for *C. neoformans* strains (Voelz et al., 2009). In addition to replication, yeasts can be expulsed from macrophages by a non-lytic mechanism that leaves both *C. neoformans* and macrophages intact and capable of replication and growth (Alvarez and Casadevall, 2006; Ma et al., 2006; Alvarez and Casadevall, 2007; Johnston and May, 2010). *C. neoformans* can also be phagocytosed by activated neutrophils (Kozel et al., 1987). The capsule of *C. neoformans* induces neutrophils to release proinflammatory cytokines, such as IL-1β, IL-6, IL-8 and TNF-α (Retini et al., 1996). Neutrophils can kill *C. neoformans* by non-oxidative mechanisms, including neutrophil defensins and calprotectin (Mambula et al., 2000). Interestingly, induction of neutropenia in mouse models of infection reduces their susceptibility to infection (Mednick et al., 2003).

Although innate immune responses against *Rhizopus,* the main causative agent of mucormycosis, have not yet been fully characterized, recent work has shown that *Rhizopus* can trigger a common innate sensing pathway in DCs that leads to the production of IL-23 and drives Th17-type responses (Chamilos et al., 2010). This is due to interaction of dectin -1 with β-glucans on the surface of *Rhizopus* hyphae.

### 3.2 NK cell activity

Another innate immune response to pulmonary fungal pathogens is due to recognition and action by natural killer (NK) cells. NK cells were thought to act primarily against viruses and tumors, but more recent studies have shown that NK cells have a wide variety of functions against bacteria, fungi, and parasites (Newman and Riley, 2007).

In *H. capsulatum* infection, there is little evidence of a protective role for NK cells. While beige mice (lacking functional NK cells) are more susceptible to *H. capsulatum* infection, T cells play a greater role in controlling infection (Patino et al., 1987). In studies evaluating both beige mice and mice depleted of NK cells, beige mice were still more susceptible to infection, while mice depleted of NK cells were no more susceptible to infection than WT mice, therefore indicating no major role for NK cells in protection (Suchyta et al., 1988). However, mice deficient in perforin, a major component of NK cell anti-microbial activity, had accelerated mortality and increased fungal burden (Zhou et al., 2001). Infection with *Coccidioides* during depletion of NK cells leads to increased susceptibility to infection (Petkus and Baum, 1987). Furthermore, NK cells have a direct cytotoxic effect on *Coccidioides* young spherule and endospore cells (Petkus and Baum, 1987). In *Paracoccidioides,* studies have shown increased NK cell activity in infected hamsters compared to uninfected controls. Impaired NK cell activity was associated with a decrease in cell-mediated immunity (CMI) and an increase in histopathologic lesions. However, after initial activation, NK cells alone were not able to control dissemination of *Paracoccidiodes* (Peracoli et al., 1995). *In vitro* NK cell activity correlated with growth inhibition of *Paracoccidiodes* yeast (Jimenez and Murphy, 1984).

In neutropenic mice with *A. fumigatus* infection, NK cells are the major cell type responsible for the production of IFN-γ early in the infection. Additionally, depletion of NK cells reduces IFN-γ levels and caused increased pulmonary fungal load (Park et al., 2009). NK cells have direct anti-fungal activity against hyphae but not against resting conidia (Schmidt et al., 2011). Killing is due to production of mediators by NK cells, including perforin. However, *A. fumigatus* can also down-regulate some cytokines induced by the NK cells, including IFN-γ and GM-CSF (Schmidt et al., 2011). In addition, recruitment of NK cells to the lung during *A. fumigatus* infection by the chemokine MCP-1 is required for optimal clearance of the organism from the lungs (Morrison et al., 2003). During *Pneumocystis* infection in SCID mice (lacking T and B cells), NK cells were responsible for production of cytokines such as IFN-γ, TNF-α, TNF-β, IL-10, and IL-12 (Warschkau et al., 1998). Recent studies have shown that NK cells are recruited to the lung during *Pneumocystis* infection and are important in fungal clearance of murine PCP (M. Kelly and J. Shellito, personal communication). Further, combined depletion of NK and $CD4^+$ T cells resulted in increased pulmonary fungal burden compared to individual depletion of each subset. In vitro, NK cells have direct microbicidal activity against *Pneumocystis*, and this anti-fungal activity is significantly enhanced in the presence of $CD4^+$ T cells, suggesting that both cell types are necessary for a protective response against *Pneumocystis* infection (M. Kelly and J. Shellito, personal communication). Early studies showed that NK cells can directly kill *C. neoformans* (Murphy and McDaniel, 1982). Further, IFN-γ production by NK cells enhances elimination of the fungus in murine models (Kawakami et al., 2001a; Kawakami et al., 2001b; Kawakami et al., 2001c). Depletion of NK cells using anti-asialo GM antibody resulted in increased fungal burden in mice (Hidore et al., 1991a; Hidore et al., 1991b). Increased fungal burden was seen in beige mice compared to wild-type mice, and in mice depleted of $NK1.1^+$ NK cells, fungal burden was also increased compared to controls (Lipscomb et al., 1987; Salkowski and Balish, 1991). Human NK cells kill *C. neoformans* (Levitz and Dupont, 1993), and this killing is enhanced in the presence of anti-cryptococcal antibodies (Miller et al., 1990). Binding of NK cells is required for cryptococcal killing, and requires disulfide bonds and is dependent on magnesium (Nabavi and Murphy, 1985; Hidore and Murphy, 1989; Murphy et al., 1991). Killing of *C. neoformans* is due to perforin interaction with the organism (Ma et al., 2004; Marr et al., 2009). In summary, NK cells act as accessory cells in antifungal host defenses contributing to clearance of fungi by a variety of mechanisms.

### 3.3 Gamma/delta T cell activity

The role of gamma delta (γδ) T cells during the immune response to pulmonary fungal pathogens is diverse. During infection with *Cryptococcus*, mice genetically deficient or depleted in γδ T cells have reduced fungal burden compared to controls. Further, mice lacking γδ T cells had increased levels of IFN-γ and decreased levels of TGF-β compared to controls, therefore suggesting that γδ T cells are detrimental to protective immunity during cryptococcal infection (Uezu et al., 2004). In *Pneumocystis* pneumonia, $CD4^+$ T cells are necessary for protection against infection, but γδ cells are known to infiltrate into the lung during pneumonia (Kagi et al., 1993; Agostini et al., 1995; Steele et al., 2002). However, resolution of pulmonary *Pneumocystis* infection is augmented in γδ T cell–deficient mice, (Steele et al., 2002), suggesting that these cells are detrimental to clearance of the organism. Further, the absence of γδ T cells led to an increase in recruitment of $CD8^+$ T cells and production of cytokines such as IFN-γ. Complete lack of all T cell subsets (αβ and γδ) during *Pneumocystis* infection led to lethal consequences (Hanano and Kaufmann, 1999). Thus, γδ T cells have either a limited role in antifungal protection or are detrimental to antifungal host defenses.

### 3.4 Innate anti-fungal defenses by non-immune cells

While innate immune cells and components of the innate immune system are the predominant innate immune defenses, it has also been shown that unconventional cells, such as epithelial cells can also play a role in anti-fungal innate host responses. Airway epithelial cells are capable of uptake and processing of antigens and initiation of Th-type immune responses (Gereke et al., 2009). *P. brasiliensis* interacts with and can be internalized by bronchial epithelial cells (Mendes-Giannini et al., 1994, and this internalization is due to activation of a tyrosine kinase pathway (Monteiro da Silva et al., 2007; Hanna et al., 2000). In addition, uptake of *P. brasiliensis* causes both cytoskeletal rearrangements as well as apoptosis of the epithelial cells (Mendes-Giannini et al., 2004). *C. neoformans* can bind to pulmonary epithelial cells by a mechanism believed to be due to carbohydrate moieties that can be a ligand for the yeast (Merkel and Scofield, 1997). *C. neoformans* interaction with bronchial epithelial cells causes the production of IL-8, but epithelial cells are also susceptible to damage by the organism (Guillot et al., 2008a). In *A. fumigatus* infection, conidia can be taken up by tracheal epithelial cells, alveolar type II cells, and endothelial cells (Paris et al., 1997). Further, cytokines such as IL-6 and IL-8 are released by epithelial cells *in vitro* following stimulation with *A. fumigatus* proteases (Borger et al., 1999) or by *A. fumigatus* hyphal fragments (Zhang et al., 2005) and nasal epithelium. And nasal epithelium can engulf *A. fumigatus* conidia (Botterel et al., 2008). Epithelial cells can also release antimicrobial peptides following stimulation with fungal organisms. Epithelial cells *in vitro* cultured with *A. fumigatus* conidia, swollen conidia, or hyphae produced large amounts of beta defensins (Alekseeva et al., 2009). Airway epithelial cells internalize *A. fumigatus* conidia, and a genome-wide analysis revealed differential gene expression in epithelial cells with conidia compared to cells without conidia. Genes that were upregulated with conidia included genes involved in repair and inflammation, such as matrix metalloproteinases and chemokines (Gomez et al., 2010). In *Pneumocystis,* several studies have shown that the organism interacts with pulmonary epithelial cells. The interaction of *Pneumocystis* with epithelial cells was shown to be one of the initial steps in infection (Lanken et al., 1980; Yoneda and Walzer, 1980; Long et al., 1986; Millard et al., 1990). The β-glucan from the *Pneumocystis* cell wall can stimulate pulmonary epithelial cells to produce IL-8, and the organism can induce the production of MCP-1 and ICAM -1 (Yu and Limper, 1997; Evans et al., 2005; Wang et al., 2007; Carmona et al., 2010). Interaction of *Pneumocystis* and alveolar epithelial cells also leads to the production of the chemokine MIP-2 following NF-κB signaling (Evans et al., 2005; Wang et al., 2005). These studies show that non-immune cells, such as epithelial cells, play a role in pulmonary anti-fungal immunity.

## 4. T cell and antibody mediated immune responses to fungal infections

### 4.1 Adaptive responses against pulmonary fungal pathogens

When challenged with pathogenic fungi, the adaptive immune system is capable of mounting an effective response against most fungal species to eliminate fungal infections and maintain immunological memory that prevents their reoccurrence. However, fungi are ubiquitous in the host's environment including the saprophytes and opportunists that survive on the host's body surfaces and thus, the adaptive immune system is constantly challenged by fungal antigens. Excessive response to these antigens could lead to allergic responses or other types of immunopathological reactions. The balance between day-to-day fungal antigen exposure and the immune system is thought to lead to a homeostatic state defined as protective tolerance. Protective tolerance allows the host to keep possible fungal pathogens "in check" while preserving integrity of the natural barriers, which are potential portals for fungal infections (Romani and Puccetti, 2008; de Luca et al., 2010a; Littman and Rudensky, 2010).

T cells are responsible for orchestration of adaptive immune responses and T cell derived signals produced in response to specific antigens lead to targeted expansion, recruitment, activation of leukocytes, and regulation of B cell antibody responses. T cells also serve as a pool of immunological memory. Additionally, T cells have been shown to directly act as the fungicidal effector cells and serve as regulators of inflammatory responses, contributing to the development and maintenance of the protective tolerance. These regulatory mechanisms are designed to limit the damage that the host immune system can inflict on host tissues during incorrect and/or excessive host responses. Thus, properly functioning T cells are responsible for building up protective immunity against fungal pathogens and play an essential role in maintaining normal homeostasis of the immune system in the context of normal presence of fungal antigens.

### 4.2 CD4$^+$ and CD8$^+$ T cell mediated immunity

The importance of T cells in antifungal protection is well documented. T-cell deficient individuals show diminished resistance to fungal infections including coccidiomycosis (Kappe et al., 1998) cryptococcosis (Kovacs et al., 1985; Chuck and Sande, 1989; Spitzer et al., 1993; Jarvis and Harrison, 2007), histoplamosis (Odio et al., 1999), pneumocystis pneumonia (Kelly and Shellito), *Paracoccidioides* (Bava et al., 1991; Brummer et al., 1993), as well as pulmonary aspergillosis (Mylonakis et al., 1998). Likewise, laboratory studies have shown a strong contribution and/or requirement of T cells for protection against most pathogenic fungi such as *Coccidioides* (Fierer et al., 2006), *Cryptococcus* (Lim and Murphy, 1980; Mody et al., 1990; Huffnagle et al., 1991; Huffnagle and Lipscomb, 1992; Mody et al., 1994), *Pneumocystis* (Harmsen and Stankiewicz, 1990), *Histoplasma* (Deepe et al., 1984), *Paracoccidioides* (Cano et al., 2000) and *Aspergillus* (Cenci et al., 1997). These epidemiological and experimental studies have established that T cells are an important component of the antifungal host resistance.

Both subsets of T lymphocytes, CD4$^+$ and CD8$^+$ cells, are involved in antifungal host defenses. CD4$^+$ T cells classically represent the T helper cell population. The T helper function was defined by MHC II restricted antigen specific activation of B-cell clones needed for the generation of specific antibodies. The CD4$^+$ cell function in cell-mediated immunity (CMI) likewise requires antigen presenting cells and MHC II restricted antigen presentation. Presentation of antigen to the reactive T cells by dendritic cells and/or macrophages results in cytokine production. Through generation of different cytokine spectra, CD4$^+$ T cells orchestrate recruitment and activation of various leukocyte subsets. The cytokines produced by the effector T cells are essential for macrophage fungicidal function and granuloma formation, but also may support chronic inflammation and immunopathology (Arora et al., 2005; Chen et al., 2008; Jain et al., 2009; Zhang et al., 2009). Thus, cytokine induction by differentially polarized T-cell lineages is the major determinant for fungicidal potential of distal effector cells. Although the effector CD4$^+$ cell function relies predominantly on cytokine production, CD4$^+$ T-cells are capable of fungal killing via direct cell contact. At least in some biological circumstances, the direct fungicidal effect of CD4$^+$ T cells relies on granulysin as the fungicidal mediator (Zheng et al., 2007; Zheng et al., 2008).

In contrast with CD4$^+$ T cells, CD8$^+$ T cells are classically viewed as cytotoxic lymphocytes. These cells respond to antigen presentation in the context of MHC I, to enable their cytotoxic machinery. Such cytotoxic responses are particularly crucial in responses to viral infection and tumor cells, leading to elimination of the virally infected or tumor-transformed cells by cytotoxic lymphocytes. CD8+ cells also play an important role in host defenses to bacterial, parasitic and fungal infections (Oykhman and Mody, 2010). Numerous studies showed that CD8+ T cells significantly contribute to protection against *Cryptococcus, Pneumocystis, Histoplasma* and *Blastomyces*, even in the absence of CD4+ T cells. Depending on the type and virulence of the fungal pathogen, CD8+ cells could afford either partial or a complete protection against the major fungal pathogens in experimental models. In this context, CD8+ T cells could induce all the protective effector functions of CD4+ T cells including production of protective cytokines. Another important aspect of CD8+ T cell effector function is the direct fungicidal effect of CD8+ T cells. Such direct fungicidal activity of CD8+ T cells have been demonstrated for *C. neoformans* (Ma et al., 2002). The killing of *C. neoformans* requires direct cell contact; it is enhanced by IL-15 and is thought to be mediated by granulysin. The direct cytotoxic effects are most pronounced when lymphocytes from fungus-immunized mice are used, however, a relatively high rate of binding of T cells to the fungus suggests that these cytotoxic mechanisms are innate rather than adaptive.

### 4.3 Immune polarization in antifungal host defenses

T helper cell subsets characterized by differential cytokine production by differentially programmed T-cell lineages were initially defined as Th1 and Th2 (Mosmann et al., 1986; Cherwinski et al., 1987). The types of immune responses driven by each of these cell lineages are described as Th1 and Th2 immune responses, generate different types of immune effector responses, and show different spectra of effectiveness against different classes of pathogens. For effective control/clearance of the majority of fungal pathogens, Th1 is the required type of the immune response. The Th1 response is promoted by IL-12, IFN-γ, and TNF-α. The two latter cytokines are also the major products of Th1 helper T cells (Cherwinski et al., 1987). Th1-type T-cells are responsible for the delayed-type hypersensitivity (DTH) reactions and CMI associated with vigorous proinflammatory responses and granuloma formation (Cher and Mosmann, 1987) and induction of IgG2a class antibodies in B cells (Stevens et al., 1988). The Th2 immune response is characterized by T-cell production of IL-4, IL-5, IL-9, IL-10, and IL-13 (Cherwinski et al., 1987), IgG1 and IgE antibody production by B cells (Stevens et al., 1988) and the presence of eosinophilic inflammation (Huffnagle et al., 1994; Cenci et al., 1999; Olszewski et al., 2001). The Th1 and Th2 responses counter-regulate each other predominantly via an IL-4/IFN-γ negative feedback loop (Fernandez-Botran et al., 1988; Gajewski and Fitch, 1988); however other cytokines can be also involved in Th1/Th2 regulation. The oversimplified Th1/Th2 paradigm has further evolved as new T cell lineages were defined. Th17 and regulatory type T cells (Treg), are T-cell lineages that are distinct from Th1 and Th2 cells that possess distinct functions in host defenses. Th17 cells are generated following the priming with IL-6 and TGF-β and sustained by the presence of IL-23. Th17 cells classically produce IL-17 and IL-22, however, a subset of Th17 cells can produce IFN-γ. Regulatory T-cells are thought to be responsible for tolerance that prevents auto-immune diseases and to contribute to resolution of inflammatory responses. These effects of Tregs are thought to be mediated by anti-inflammatory cytokines IL-10 and TGF-β, which are signature cytokines for Treg cells. New Th-cell lineages continue to be described including Th22 (Eyerich et al., 2009; Fujita et al., 2009) and Th9 (Soroosh and Doherty, 2009). Just like CD4+ effector T-cells, CD8+ T cells can also display a polarization pattern and thus can be an important source of the polarizing cytokines. Thus, both CD4+ and CD8+ T cells contribute to the cytokine balance during the immune response (Huffnagle et al., 1994).

### 4.4 Th1/2/17/22 cytokine responses

The protective role of Th1 along with the requirement of type 1 cytokines for fungal clearance have been demonstrated in models of cryptococcosis (Huffnagle et al., 1994; Kawakami et al., 1997; Blackstock et al., 1999; Abe et al., 2000; Traynor et al., 2000; Olszewski et al., 2001; Herring et al., 2002; Arora et al., 2005; Hernandez et al., 2005; Lindell et al., 2006; Wormley et al., 2007; Chen et al., 2008; Guillot et al., 2008b; Jain et al., 2009; Wozniak et al., 2009; Zhang et al., 2009), *Coccidioides* (Silva and Benitez, 2005), *Paracocidioides* (Cano et al., 1998), *Histoplama* (Zhou et al., 1995; Deepe and Gibbons, 2006) and *Blastomyces* (Brummer et al., 2006) infections. Th1 skewing is beneficial for clearance of *Aspergillus* (Cenci et al., 1997), although clearance of the filamentous fungi is mainly a domain of the innate immune system. The Th1 cytokine environment promotes clearance of fungi by supporting the classical activation of macrophages (Mantovani et al., 2001). Pathogenic fungi possess mechanisms that interfere with their recognition by macrophages. These fungi can survive within macrophage unless additional "external" stimulation occurs to activate fungicidal mechanisms. Such stimulation can be provided by Th1-type cytokines, especially IFN-γ (Arora et al., 2005; Hardison et al.). In the context of a Th1 immune response, macrophages become classically activated and abundantly generate fungicidal molecules such as nitric oxide produced by nitric oxide synthase, an enzyme that utilizes L-arginine. Importance of classical macrophage activation and production of nitric oxide for fungal clearance has been demonstrated for *Blastomyces* (Brummer et al., 2005; Kethineni et al., 2006), *Cryptococcus* (Granger et al., 1990; Alspaugh and Granger, 1991; Rivera et al., 2002; Arora et al., 2005; Zhang et al.; Hardison et al.), *Histoplasma* (Zhou et al., 1995; Allendoerfer and Deepe, 1998; Allen and Deepe, 2006) and *Paracocidiodes* (Moreira et al.; Pinzan et al.) infections. The deficiencies in cytokines that support classical activation of macrophages GM-CSF, IFN-γ, TNF-α, IL-12 are generally associated with the development of progressive fungal infection (Romani et al., 1994; Kawakami et al., 1999; Rayhane et al., 1999; Herring et al., 2005; Deepe and Gibbons, 2006) consistent with the general conclusion that Th1-type immune responses and type 1 cytokines are most optimal for resistance against fungal infections.

Unlike Th1-type responses, the Th2 response is non-protective and frequently results in pathological responses to fungal challenges. For most fungal species, Th2 responses and type 2 cytokines decrease clearance of fungus. This is attributed to: 1) a suppression of protective Th1 responses due to a mutual counterregulatory feedback loop (Cenci et al., 1999) and 2) a generation of alternatively activated macrophages that can harbor fungal organisms (Arora et al., 2005; Jain et al., 2009; Osterholzer et al., 2009a; Zhang et al., 2009). Th2 cytokines such as IL-4, IL-13 are the major trigger of alternative activation of macrophages (Arora et al., 2005; Jain et al., 2009; Zhang et al., 2009). These alternatively activated macrophages do not express nitric oxide synthase but induce arginase which metabolizes L-arginine without yielding fungicidal nitric oxide. In the Th2 biased experimental models of fungal infections, intracellular survival of fungus within macrophages parallels high induction of alternatively activated macrophage markers (Arora et al., 2005; Zhang et al., 2009; Hardison et al.).

Increased production of Th2-type cytokines has been associated with increased susceptibility to *Cryptococcus* (Arora et al., 2005; Zhang et al., 2009; Hardison et al.) and *Paracoccidioides* (Ruas et al., 2009) infections and to invasive pulmonary aspergillosis (Cenci et al., 1997; Cenci et al., 1999). Fungus-triggered Th2-type responses in the respiratory system may also lead to allergic diseases such rhinitis/sinusitis, asthma, allergic bronchopulmonary mycosis. Th2 type responses are highly detrimental to the respiratory system by promoting mucus hypersecretion/goblet cell metaplasia, eosinophilic inflammation, and peribronchial fibrosis all of which contribute to impaired airway function. Cytokines IL-4, IL-5 and IL-13 are the major triggers of these pathologies as increased expression of these cytokines can be reproduced along with the allergic symptoms in the lungs challenged with fungi or their antigenic components (Blease et al., 2000; Arora et al., 2005; Jain et al., 2009; Zhang et al., 2009). Some of the fungal antigens can directly promote Th2 skewing. The secreted protein fraction from *Aspergillus fumigatus* promotes Th2 bias of the immune response (Bozza et al., 2009). Th2 pathologies are also found in mouse models of *C. neoformans* infections (Abe et al., 2000; Jain et al., 2009; Osterholzer et al., 2009b) (Figure 1). Expression of enzymes phospholipase B and urease by *C. neoformans* promote Th2 bias in the infected mice (Noverr et al., 2003; Osterholzer et al., 2009b). While Th2-biased responses are clearly undesirable in most types of fungal infections the exception is *Pneumocystis* infection, in which the Th2 response can contribute to fungal clearance (Shellito et al., 2000; McKinley et al., 2006; Hu et al., 2009).

Figure 1.

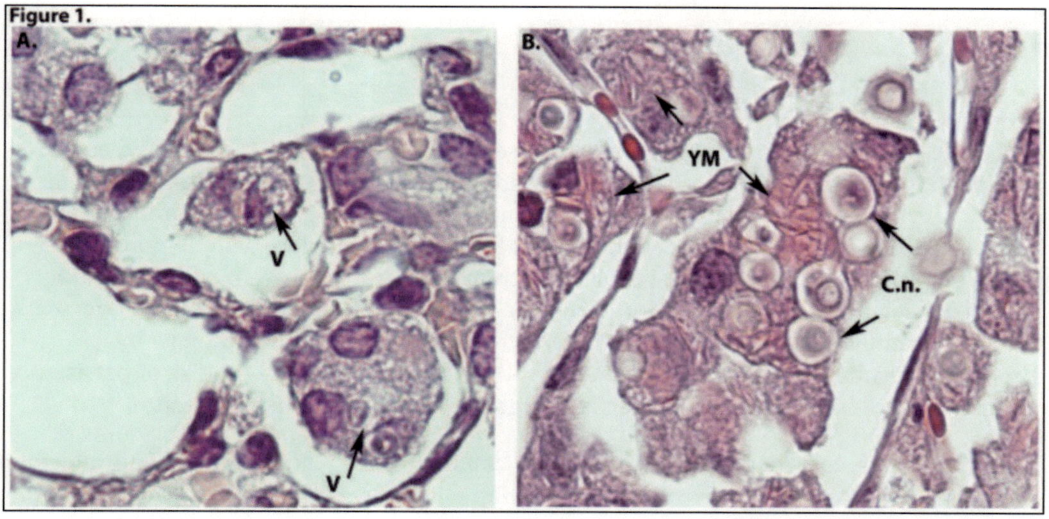


Fig. 1. Classical versus alternative activation of macrophages during pulmonary infection with *C. neoformans*. A) Classically activated macrophages upregulate fungicidal mechanisms that eliminate ingested fungi. Note that ingested intracellular organisms show signs of degradation. B) Alternatively activated macrophages (AAM) harbor the ingested fungi. Note the abundant capsule formation (evidence of fungal metabolic activity) and dividing organisms (evidence of intracellular growth) within AAM. Alternative activation of macrophages is associated with crystallization of chitinase family proteins YM1 and YM2, a hallmark of AAM-induced pathology. **V**-vacuoles with the remnants of destroyed organisms, **YM**- YM1/YM2 crystals, **C.n.** - intact cryptococcal organisms.

The effects of Th17 responses and the IL-17 cytokine family in anti-fungal host responses may be protective or non-protective depending on fungal species and sites of infection (Figure 2). Thus, Th17 responses may be beneficial for some types of fungal infections or

**Figure 2.**

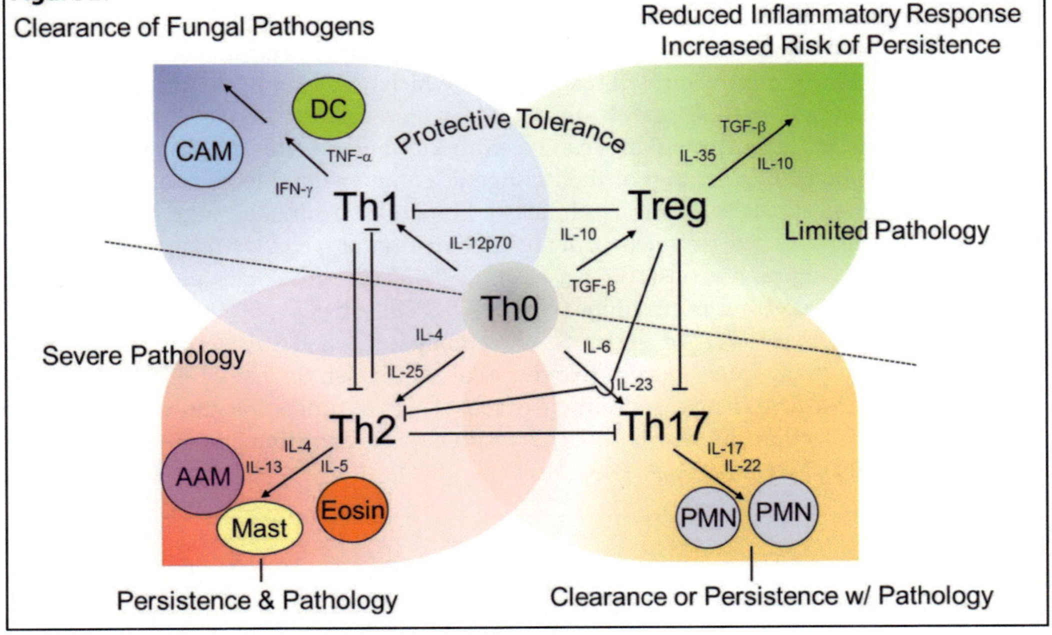


Fig. 2. Th polarization in antifungal host defenses. The outcome of Th1, Th2, Th17, and Treg polarization results from balance between Th lineages which can mutually regulate each other via cytokine feedback loops. Resultant outcome can either promote clearance of the fungal infection or result in persistent infection and limited or severe pathology. Th1 response promotes control of most fungal infections; Th2 leads to severe pathology and fungal persistence; Th17 may support clearance or persistence of different fungal infections, but may promote chronic neutrophilic inflammation. Treg may limit pathology by promoting resolution of the inflammatory response, but may increase the risk of persistence. Correct balance between Th1 and Treg is thought to support protective tolerance.

exhibit detrimental effects. In the *H. capsulatum* infection model, IL-17 neutralization increases pulmonary fungal burden in connection with increased Treg numbers, suggesting that Th17 is beneficial for clearance of *Histoplasma* (Kroetz and Deepe, 2010). Th17 responses also contribute to anticryptococcal protection and the development of the protective inflammatory response in *C. neoformans* infected lungs (Zhang et al., 2009; Hardison et al., 2010b; Wozniak et al., 2011a).

The IL-23/IL-17 axis contributes to clearance of *Pneumocystis* (Rudner et al., 2007). However, in IFN-γ deficient mice infected with *Pneumocystis* the development of strong Th17 response is detrimental, suggesting that a balance between IFN-γ and IL-17 is needed for optimal clearance of *Pneumocystis* (Hu et al., 2009). At other mucosal sites, the effects of Th17 are variable. Th17 cells and IL-17 receptor signaling are required for mucosal host defenses in oral candidiasis (Conti et al., 2009); whereas Th17 impairs antifungal resistance and promotes inflammation in gastric infection model (Zelante et al., 2007). Th17 responses impair antifungal resistance and promotes inflammatory damage in the lungs of mice infected with *Aspergillus* (Zelante et al., 2007; Bozza et al., 2009; D'Angelo et al., 2009).

Overall, the Th17 response may have beneficial effects for clearance of some fungal pathogens; however it also has high potential to produce undesirable effects, including inflammatory damage.

Excessive immune reaction and uncontrolled inflammation can result in serious damage of the inflicted organs and tissues. Anti-inflammatory or regulatory cytokines such as IL-10 and TGF-β are an important part of the balance which prevents over exuberant inflammation during acute responses. These cytokines are also thought to be important components of resolution and tissue repair that occurs after elimination of the pathogen. Regulatory T cells are important sources of these cytokines and their role in inflammatory diseases and in the maintenance of healthy tissue homeostasis becomes increasingly appreciated (Romani and Puccetti, 2008; De Luca et al., 2010b; Littman and Rudensky, 2010). The importance of balance between pro-inflammatory processes and Treg cell regulation has recently been demonstrated in models of *Pneumocystis* (McKinley et al., 2006) and *Histoplasma* infections (Kroetz and Deepe). The excessive/damaging inflammatory reaction can be exemplified by immune reconstitution inflammatory syndrome (IRIS). IRIS is characterized by uncontrolled inflammatory responses with high induction of IFN-γ, TNF-α and other pro-inflammatory cytokines (Mori and Levin, 2009). Overproduction of these cytokines, rather than having protective effects, contributes to tissue injury that leads to worsening of the patient condition and high mortality (Mori and Levin, 2009). Interestingly, occurrence of IRIS in HIV patients who undergo antiretroviral therapy is particularly high in patients with *Cryptococcus* and *Pneumocystis* infections (Singh et al., 2005; Singh and Perfect, 2007; Murdoch et al., 2008). The mechanism of inadequate inflammatory response in IRIS is not understood, however it has been proposed that the regulatory mechanisms that control the inflammation, including Tregs are not sufficiently mobilized to put a break on this inflammatory response (McKinley et al., 2006; Shankar et al., 2008). In fact, patients with IRIS showed reduced suppressor function and diminished secretion of anti-inflammatory IL-10 by Tregs in one of the studies (Seddiki et al., 2009). Tregs are critical for maintaining the proper homeostasis in the GI track, and such mechanisms of protective tolerance are likely to be critical in the respiratory tract which is constantly exposed to inhaled fungal antigens. Insufficiency of the regulatory mechanisms most likely contributes to the development of allergic diseases. Thus, Tregs cells are important for maintaining balance between appropriate clearance rate and the inflammatory tissue damage. Such balance can be disturbed and the excessive Treg function may promote fungal persistence. A detrimental role of IL-10 has been demonstrated in cryptococcal infection models (Blackstock et al., 1999; Arora et al., 2005). Future studies will be needed to evaluate the possible role of Tregs in fungal infections, especially in the patients who develop mycoses without apparent immunodeficiency.

The polarization of T cells to Th1, Th2, Th17 and Treg lineages is important for the development of protective immunity, protective tolerance, chronic/allergic syndromes, or overwhelming allergic reactions. The proper balance maintained by the mutual regulation between these arms of the immune system is necessary to optimize clearance and minimize inflammatory damage to the infected tissues in the context of fungal infection. Our present understanding of these responses evolved from an oversimplified polarized Th1/Th2 paradigm to a broader understanding of mutual regulation ongoing during the immune process. Recent studies show that the Th1, Th2, Th17 responses co-exist in a fungus infected lungs and the balance of cytokine production alters during different time points in a chronic fungal infection (Arora et al., 2011). Modulation of these responses can be achieved experimentally and therapeutically by use of cytokines and vaccination with different fractions of fungal antigens resulting in the induction of the proper and protective Th-cell polarization.

### 4.5 Vaccine-induced therapies targeting cellular mediated immunity

Currently, there are no standardized vaccines available for the prevention of fungal diseases in humans (as discussed earlier). A preponderance of evidence points to the development of cell-mediated immune responses, principally by Th1–type CD4+ T cells, as the predominant host defense mechanism against primary and opportunistic pulmonary fungal pathogens (Cutler et al., 2007). Further, ablation or neutralization of several Th1-type cytokines renders mice more susceptible to experimental infection with a number of fungal pathogens. Consequently, there has been great interest in identifying antigens that elicit protective CMI against fungal infections; some of which will be discussed herein.

Vaccination with native or recombinant Hsp60 from *H. capsulatum* or a domain within Hsp60 conferred protection in mice given a sub-lethal challenge with yeast cells and prolonged survival in mice given a lethal challenge (Gomez et al., 1995; Deepe and Gibbons, 2002). Protection was CD4+ T cell dependent and associated with the induction of IFN-γ, IL-12 and, surprisingly, the Th2-type cytokine IL-10 (Deepe and Gibbons, 2002; Scheckelhoff and Deepe, 2005). A similar vaccination strategy in mice using Hsp70 did not induce robust IL-12 or IFN-γ responses and protection against subsequent challenge with live yeast. Neutralization of IL-12 or IFN-γ abolished the protective efficacy of the Hsp60 vaccine in mice further highlighting the importance of these Th1-type cytokines in the induction of protection against *H. capsulatum*.

Similarly, vaccination of mice with recombinant Hsp60 derived from *P. brasiliensis* elicited protection against a lethal intranasal challenge with yeast (de Bastos Ascenco Soares et al., 2008). The protective effect of *P. basiliensis* Hsp60 was abrogated following the depletion of CD4+ T cells or neutralization of IFN-γ; similar to that observed for Hsp60 from *H. capsulatum* (Scheckelhoff and Deepe, 2005; de Bastos Ascenco Soares et al., 2008). However, IL-10 was not produced following antigen stimulation of splenocytes obtained from *P. basiliensis* Hsp60 immunized mice. While the efficacy of vaccination with forms of Hsp60 from *H. capsulatum* and *P. brasiliensis* are encouraging, immunization with recombinant Hsp60 derived from *C. immitis* resulted in predominantly Th2 cytokine responses and little protection against a subsequent intraperitoneal challenge (Li et al., 2001). Thus, the induction of Th1-type immune responses in the lungs appears critical for the development of protection following immunization with Hsp60.

Evaluation of live attenuated, recombinant, and DNA vaccines of *C. immitis* in murine models have also highlighted the importance of Th1-type cytokine production, particularly IFN-γ, in protection against this microbe (reviewed in (Cole et al., 2004; Cox and Magee, 2004; Xue et al., 2009)). Mice immunized with recombinant aspartyl protease (Pep1), alpha-mannosidase (Amn1), or phospholipase B (Plb) individually or together as amultivalent vaccine experienced a significant reduction in fungal burden and prolonged survival against a lethal pulmonary challenge with C. *posadasii* arthroconidia compared to controls (Tarcha et al., 2006). Approximately 85% of mice immunized with the multivalent recombinant vaccine survived to day 90 post-inoculation. Similarly, immunization of mice with two recombinant antigens, *Coccidiodes*-specific antigen (CSA) and the proline-rich cell wall protein Ag2/PRA, either as a mixture of two separately expressed proteins or as a single chimeric expression product was shown to protect mice from a lethal intranasal infection with C. *posadasii* (Shubitz et al., 2006). The protection observed with each vaccination strategy was associated with robust IFN-γ responses in protected mice, again showing the importance of Th1-type cytokines during protective host responses. Further, these studies highlighted the utility of a multivalent vaccination strategy that potentially evokes protective responses towards a broader set of T-cell epitopes.

The importance of $CD4^+$ T cells and the generation of Th1-type responses towards eliciting protection against pulmonary fungal pathogens are also observed in vaccination models using a live *C. neoformans* strain engineered to express IFN-γ (Wormley et al., 2007) (Wozniak et al., 2009) (Young et al., 2009), a live attenuated strain of *B. dermatitidis* (Wuthrich et al., 2000), and recombinant *A. fumigatus* protein Asp f3 (Diaz-Arevalo et al., 2011). Immunization with recombinant Asp f3 of *A. fumigatus* protected cortisone acetate immune suppressed mice from an experimental pulmonary infection with *A. fumigatus* conidia (Diaz-Arevalo et al., 2011). The protection was dependent on $CD4^+$ T cells as their depletion reduced the survival of vaccinated mice and adoptive transfer of Aspf3 primed $CD4^+$ T cells into non-vaccinated mice enhanced their survival against experimentally induced pulmonary aspergillosis. Generation of sterilizing immunity in mice following pulmonary immunization with a *C. neoformans* strain engineered to express murine IFN-γ, designated H99γ, was shown to require the induction of Th1-type cell-mediated immune responses (Wozniak et al., 2009). Interestingly, B-cell deficient mice immunized with H99γ were protected from a subsequent lethal pulmonary challenge with WT *C. neoformans* (Wozniak et al., 2009; Young et al., 2009; Wozniak et al., 2011b). Also, vaccination of mice with an attenuated strain of *B. dermatitidis* containing a targeted deletion in the *BAD1* locus resulted in prolonged survival that was chiefly mediated by IFN-γ and TNF-α production by $CD4^+$ T cells (Wuthrich et al., 2000; Wuthrich et al., 2002). Although these studies show that Th1-type $CD4^+$ T cell responses are required for optimal host responses against these pulmonary pathogens, studies in *H. capsulatum, B. dermititidis*, and *C. neoformans* highlight the inherent plasticity of the host response against pulmonary fungal pathogens. That is that some elements of the immune response can compensate for the loss of other components.

Vaccine-induced immunity against *B. dermatitidis* was shown be mediated by $CD4^+$ α/β T cell production of TNF-α and IFN-γ (Wuthrich et al., 2002). Moreover, the initiation, but not maintenance, of protective memory responses to *B dermatitidis* required IL-12 production (Wuthrich et al., 2005). However, vaccine-induced immunity could be elicited and expressed in IFN-γ and TNF-α deficient mice. The reciprocal cytokine or the presence of GM-CSF was shown to compensate for the loss of IFN-γ and TNF-α showing some plasticity in the vaccine-induced host response to *Blastomyces* (Wuthrich et al., 2002). Furthermore, a role for Th17 cells in vaccine-induced protection against multiple pulmonary fungal pathogens has been shown (Wuthrich et al., 2011). Specifically, protection afforded by vaccination against *C. posadassi, H. capsulatum*, and *B. dermatitidis* was observed to be dependent on IL-17. In fact, IL-17 was shown to be indispensable since vaccinated IL-17A or IL-17RA deficient mice showed impaired anti-fungal resistance despite having normal Th1-type cytokine expression. In contrast, IL-17A was shown to contribute to but ultimately be dispensable for protection against experimental pulmonary cryptococcosis in *C. neoformans* strain H99γ vaccinated mice (Hardison et al., 2010b; Wozniak et al., 2011a). Still, it appears imperative that vaccines strategies to prevent pulmonary mycoses be evaluated for their capacity to induce Th1 and Th17-type cytokine responses.

The induction of T cell-mediated immune responses is critical for optimal protection against pulmonary fungal pathogens (Cutler et al., 2007). Consequently, it may seem counterintuitive to suggest that vaccines designed to prevent fungal infections in patients with T cell deficiencies is possible. Nonetheless, vaccination studies using experimental models of *H. capsulatum* (Deepe and Gibbons, 2002), *P. brasiliensis* (de Bastos Ascenco Soares et al., 2008), *H. capsulatum* (Wuthrich et al., 2003), *B. dermatitidis* (Wuthrich et al., 2002; Wuthrich et al., 2003), *C. immitis* (Fierer et al., 2006), *and C. neoformans* (Wozniak et al., 2011b) have indicated that vaccine-induced protective immune responses can be elicited in immune deficient hosts. Cumulatively, the studies show that the presence of $CD4^+$ or $CD8^+$ T cells is essential for the induction (the period following vaccination) and expression (immune response following challenge) phases of the protective immune response. Protection is not induced in mice that are T cell deficient or depleted of both $CD4^+$ and $CD8^+$ T cell populations. Further, protection is lost in vaccinated mice following deletion of both T cell subsets. Interestingly, 80% of mice vaccinated with *C. neoformans* strain H99γ and subsequently depleted of both $CD4^+$ and $CD8^+$ T cells were protected from a lethal pulmonary challenge with WT *C. neoformans* (Wozniak et al., 2011b). These studies highlight dynamic compensatory mechanisms that mediate vaccine-induced protection during both the induction and expression phases of the anti-fungal immune response. Altogether, the results demonstrating the plasticity of the vaccine-induced immune response to pulmonary fungal pathogens are particularly exciting as they highlight the potential for inducing protection in immune competent and immune compromised hosts.

### 4.6 Antibody-mediated immunity and therapeutics

The contribution of antibody mediated immunity (AMI) towards protecting individuals against pulmonary fungal infections remains uncertain. Individuals with humoral deficiencies such as autosomal hyper-IgM syndrome and IgA deficiency do not exhibit an increased susceptibility to fungal infections (reviewed in Antachopoulos, 2007, 2010). In contrast, patients with X-linked hyper IgM syndrome and common-variable immunodeficiency which are often accompanied by defects in T CMI have a higher risk of developing pulmonary and invasive fungal infections like cryptococcosis and histoplasmosis. The efficacious role for antibodies during the host immune responses against fungi is like that observed against bacterial and viral pathogens. Antibodies produced in response to fungal infection serve as opsonins to promote phagocytosis, participate in antibody-dependent cellular cytotoxicity, augment Th1-type polarization, help to eliminate immunosuppressive polysaccharide antigen from serum and tissues, inhibit biofilm formation, have direct antifungal activity, and modulate the immune response to prevent host damage (reviewed in Alvarez and Casadevall, 2007; reviewed in Zaragoza and Casadevall, 2004).

Most studies showing the efficacy of AMI against pulmonary fungal pathogens has involved experimental models of PcP and cryptocococcosis. The polysaccharide capsule of *Cryptococcus*, its main virulence determinant, is predominantly comprised of the polysaccharides glucuronoxylomannan (GXM) and galactoxylomannan (GalXM) and to a much lesser extent, <1%, mannoproteins (MP) (reviewed in Zaragoza et al., 2009). Conjugate vaccines consisting of GXM combined to either tetanus toxoid (TT) or *Pseudomonas aeruginosa* exoprotein A (rEPA) induce high antibody titers (Devi et al., 1991; Casadevall et al., 1992), enhanced antifungal activity of murine and human phagocytes (Mukherjee et al., 1995c; Zhong and Pirofski, 1996, 1998) and conferred some protection against cryptococcosis in mice (Devi, 1996; Fleuridor et al., 1998; Nussbaum et al., 1999). Unfortunately, the profound suppressive effects on immune responses induced by cryptococcal polysaccharides and the highly variable immune responses observed in response to the intact GXM portion of the conjugate vaccine renders it an unlikely choice for future vaccine development (reviewed in Zaragoza et al., 2009; reviewed in Pirofski, 2001). A strategy using small peptide mimotopes (peptides which are able to induce antibodies that are capable of binding to the native antigen when administered as an immunogen) that mimic defined GXM epitopes was attempted to elicit protective antibody responses where using total GXM was unsuccessful. Zhang et al. described a peptide mimetic (P13) of GXM that was recognized by human anti-GXM antibodies (Zhang et al., 1997) and showed that vaccination with P13-protein conjugates in mice resulted in prolonged survival after a lethal *C. neoformans* challenge compared to controls (Fleuridor et al., 2001) or following establishment of a chronic infection (Datta et al., 2008).

Casadevall et al. developed a murine monoclonal antibody (MAb), 18B7, to *C. neoformans* polysaccharide that underwent phase I clinical studies in $HIV^+$ patients with cryptococcal antigenemia (Casadevall et al., 1998). A modest reduction in serum cryptococcal antigen titers was observed in patients receiving singular doses of 1 and 2 mg/kg up to 10 weeks post-treatment before returning to baseline (Casadevall et al., 1998). To date, no follow-up clinical studies have been published. A new approach using MAb 18B7 currently being investigated in mice involves conjugation of the MAb to the therapeutic radioisotopes $^{188}$Rhenium or $^{213}$Bismuth (Dadachova et al., 2003; Bryan et al., 2010). Studies have shown that administration of radiolabeled MAb 18B7 to lethally infected mice results in prolonged survival, reduced organ fungal burden, and was a more effective therapy compared to mice treated with amphotericin B. Radioimmunotherapy can be applied using MAb derived against multiple pulmonary fungal pathogens and thus may evolve into an attractive option for the treatment of other pulmonary mycoses. Lastly, while most studies have examined passive administration with antibodies targeting *C. neoformans* polysaccharide, other cryptococcal targets for passive antibody therapy under experimental investigation include melanin (Rosas et al., 2001), β-glucan (Rachini et al., 2007), heat shock protein (HSP) 90 (Nooney et al., 2005) and glucosylceramide (Rodrigues et al., 2007).

Mice deficient in B cells, either due to a targeted disruption of the IgM constant region (μMT mice) or using depletion antibodies, are more susceptible to PcP infection (Harmsen and Stankiewicz, 1991; Marcotte et al., 1996) (Lund et al., 2003; Lund et al., 2006). These studies showed that B cells were able to provide protection against PcP not only by producing Ab but also by amplifying the $CD4^+$ T cell-mediated immune response. Passive administration of an IgM mAb shown to be directed against a surface antigen present on rat-, rabbit-, ferret-, and human-derived *P. carinii* induced partial protection against PcP in animal models (Gigliotti and Hughes, 1988). Subsequent studies showed that the passive administration of mAbs recognizing kexin-like molecule (KEX1) via the intranasal route prior to experimentally induced PcP resulted in a significant reduction in pulmonary fungal burden (~99%) (Gigliotti et al., 2002).

Contrasting studies have shown that B cell deficient μMT mice have lower pulmonary fungal burden following intranasal infection with *A. fumigatus* (Montagnoli et al., 2003) or *B. dermatitidis* (Wuthrich et al., 2000) and are not more susceptible to experimental pulmonary histoplasmosis infection (Allendorfer et al., 1999) compared to WT controls. Also, passive transfer of polyclonal serum or MAbs obtained from *A. fumigatus, B. dermatitidis,* or *C. immttis* vaccinated mice did not enhance protection against a subsequent intranasal challenge with these pathogens (Kong et al., 1965; Beaman et al., 1977; Frosco et al., 1994; Wuthrich et al., 2000; Beaman et al., 1979). The role of antibodies in the host defense against fungal infection remains controversial because of its complexity. The current consensus is that antifungal antibodies can mediate protective, nonprotective, or disease-enhancing effects on host defenses during infection (Mukherjee et al., 1995a; Mukherjee et al., 1995b; Yuan et al., 1998a). Thus, resistance to disease may depend upon the proportion of protective antifungal antibodies produced during infection. In support of this concept, non-protective and protective MAbs to *C. neoformans* has been described (Mukherjee et al., 1995a; Maitta et al., 2004). Also, Nosanchuk et al. demonstrated that mice passively administered MAbs targeting a histone H2B-like protein on the surface of *H. capsulatum* before infection experienced a reduction in fungal burden and prolonged survival (Nosanchuk et al., 2003). These studies were somewhat surprising in light of previous studies showing no increased susceptibility to experimental histoplasmosis infection in B cell deficient mice (Allendorfer et al., 1999). Studies in *C. neoformans* has shown that the efficacy of MAbs appears to be dependent on several variables including host genetics (Rivera and Casadevall, 2005), Ab isotype (Yuan et al., 1995; Yuan et al., 1998b), T cell function (Yuan et al., 1997), and the presence of Th1- and Th2-related cytokines (Beenhouwer et al., 2001). AMI during the protective response to pulmonary fungal pathogens is broad and divergent, but it is clear that specific antibodies are efficacious for the host in the resolution of infection.

Studies also support the potential of using antibodies that target antigens common among multiple fungi to mediate cross-protection. Passive immunization using anti β-glucan MAbs or vaccination with β-glucan (laminarin) conjugated with the genetically-inactivated diphtheria toxin CRM197 (Lam-CRM vaccine) has been shown to confer protection against *C. neoformans, C. albicans and A. fumigatus* (Torosantucci et al., 2005; Rachini et al., 2007). Since β-glucans are found in the cell wall of fungi, the efficacy of anti-β-glucan antibodies can be very broad. Cenci et al. used a killer anti-idiotype MAb reacting to a yeast killer toxin to protect mice from a lethal *A. fumigatus* challenge during experimental bone marrow transplantation (Cenci and Romani and 2375). Killer toxin is also expressed by multiple fungal species. Mycograb (NeuTec Pharman plc.), a recombinant antibody targeting an epitope within the HSP90 of *Candida albicans* that is conserved with the corresponding protein in *C. neoformans*, has been shown to act in adjunct with amphotericin B against multiple *Candida* species and *C. neoformans*. Altogether, these studies highlight the possibility that antibodies targeting "universal' antigens common to multiple fungal species such as β-glucans, killer toxins, or Hsps may extend protection to multiple disparate fungal pathogens. Casadevall and Pirofski has published an elegant commentary on the emergence of cross-protective targets for fungi (Casadevall and Pirofski, 2007).

## 5. Conclusion

The principal route of entry for several of the primary and opportunistic fungal pathogens is via inhalation of infectious propagules into the lungs. Consequently, exposure to these fungi is unavoidable. Nevertheless, most encounters are asymptomatic due to the quick resolution of the fungi by resident effector cells within the lung. On those occasions that the fungal insult cannot be quickly eradicated, T cells, predominantly $CD4^{+}$ T cells, preside over orchestrating the adaptive responses and provide help for antibody production. T cell responses are also influenced by cytokine production by innate effector cells. Nonetheless, T cells mediate various cellular responses at the sites of infection and are ultimately responsible for either resolution or pathological reactions associated with these infections. Furthermore, T cells are important players in homeostasis and protecting integrity of natural barriers. Recent advances in experimental animal models support the premise that anti-fungal vaccines may be effective in immune compromised hosts. The efficacy of anti-fungal vaccines in immune compromised populations is undoubtedly due to the inherent plasticity of host immunity. Altogether, it is clear that immune responses to pulmonary fungal infections are as diverse as the fungi themselves but that significant ground has been made towards its understanding.

## 6. Acknowledgments

We would like to acknowledge support by grants RO1 AI071752-04 and R21 AI083718-02 from the National Institute of Allergy and Infectious Diseases (NIAID) of the National Institutes of Health (NIH) (F.L.W.Jr.) and from the US Army Research Office of the Department of Defense Contract No. W911NF-11-1-0136 (F.L.W.Jr.), and the Department of Veteran's Biomedical R&D Grant (M.A.O.). The content is solely the responsibility of the authors and does not necessarily represent the official views of NIAID of the National Institutes of Health, the Department of Defense or the Department of Veteran's affairs. The authors declare no conflicts of interest.

## 7. References

Abe K, Kadota J, Ishimatsu Y, Iwashita T, Tomono K, Kawakami K, Kohno S. 2000. Th1-Th2 cytokine kinetics in the bronchoalveolar lavage fluid of mice infected with *Cryptococcus neoformans* of different virulences. Microbiol Immunol 44:849-855.

Agostini C, Zambello R, Trentin L, Semenzato G. 1995. T lymphocytes with gamma/delta T-cell receptors in patients with AIDS and *Pneumocystis carinii* pneumonia. Aids 9:203-204.

Alekseeva L, Huet D, Femenia F, Mouyna I, Abdelouahab M, Cagna A, Guerrier D, Tichanne-Seltzer V, Baeza-Squiban A, Chermette R, Latge JP, Berkova N. 2009. Inducible expression of beta defensins by human respiratory epithelial cells exposed to *Aspergillus fumigatus* organisms. BMC Microbiol 9:33.

Allen HL, Deepe GS, Jr. 2006. B cells and CD4-CD8- T cells are key regulators of the severity of reactivation histoplasmosis. J Immunol 177:1763-1771.

Allendoerfer R, Deepe GS, Jr. 1998. Infection with *Histoplasma capsulatum*: Host-fungus interface. Rev Iberoam Micol 15:256-260.

Allendorfer R, Brunner GD, Deepe GS, Jr. 1999. Complex requirements for nascent and memory immunity in pulmonary histoplasmosis. J Immunol 162:7389-7396.

Almyroudis NG, Holland SM, Segal BH. 2005. Invasive aspergillosis in primary immunodeficiencies. Med Mycol 43 Suppl 1:S247-259.

Alspaugh JA, Granger DL. 1991. Inhibition of *Cryptococcus neoformans* replication by nitrogen oxides supports the role of these molecules as effectors of macrophage-mediated cytostasis. Infect Immun 59:2291-2296.

Alvarez M, Casadevall A. 2006. Phagosome extrusion and host-cell survival after *Cryptococcus neoformans* phagocytosis by macrophages. Curr Biol 16:2161-2165.

Alvarez M, Casadevall A. 2007. Cell-to-cell spread and massive vacuole formation after *Cryptococcus neoformans* infection of murine macrophages. BMC Immunol 8:16.

Ampel NM, Galgiani JN. 1991. Interaction of human peripheral blood mononuclear cells with *Coccidioides immitis* arthroconidia. Cell Immunol 133:253-262.

Antachopoulos C. 2010. Invasive fungal infections in congenital immunodeficiencies. Clin Microbiol Infect 16:1335-1342.

Antachopoulos C, Walsh T, Roilides E. 2007. Fungal infections in primary immunodeficiencies. Eur J Pediat 166:1099-1117.

Arora S, Hernandez Y, Erb-Downward JR, McDonald RA, Toews GB, Huffnagle GB. 2005. Role of IFN-gamma in regulating T2 immunity and the development of alternatively activated macrophages during allergic bronchopulmonary mycosis. J Immunol 174:6346-6356.

Arora S, Olszewski MA, Tsang TM, McDonald RA, Toews GB, Huffnagle GB. 2011. Effect of cytokine interplay on macrophage polarization during chronic pulmonary infection with *Cryptococcus neoformans*. Infect Immun 79:1915-1926.

Awasthi S. 2007. Dendritic cell- based vaccine against *Coccidioides* infection. Ann N Y Acad Sci.

Bauman SK, Huffnagle GB, Murphy JW. 2003. Effects of tumor necrosis factor alpha on dendritic cell accumulation in lymph nodes draining the immunization site and the impact on the anticryptococcal cell-mediated immune response. Infect Immun 71:68-74.

Bauman SK, Nichols KL, Murphy JW. 2000. Dendritic cells in the induction of protective and nonprotective anticryptococcal cell-mediated immune responses. J Immunol 165:158-167.

Bava AJ, Mistchenko AS, Palacios MF, Estevez ME, Tiraboschi NI, Sen L, Negroni R, Diez RA. 1991. Lymphocyte subpopulations and cytokine production in paracoccidioidomycosis patients. Microbiol Immunol 35:167-174.

Beaman L, Benjamini E, Pappagianis D. 1981. Role of lymphocytes in macrophage-induced killing of *Coccidioides immitis* in vitro. Infect Immun 34:347-353.

Beaman L, Benjamini E, Pappagianis D. 1983. Activation of macrophages by lymphokines: enhancement of phagosome-lysosome fusion and killing of *Coccidioides immitis*. Infect Immun 39:1201-1207.

Beaman L, Holmberg CA. 1980a. In vitro response of alveolar macrophages to infection with *Coccidioides immitis*. Infect Immun 28:594-600.

Beaman L, Holmberg CA. 1980b. Interaction of nonhuman primate peripheral blood leukocytes and *Coccidioides immitis* in vitro. Infection and immunity 29:1200-1201.

Beaman L, Pappagianis D, Benjamini E. 1977. Significance of T cells in resistance to experimental murine coccidioidomycosis. Infect Immun 17:580-585.

Beaman LV, Pappagianis D, Benjamini E. 1979. Mechanisms of resistance to infection with *Coccidioides immitis* in mice. Infect Immun 23:681-685.

Beenhouwer DO, Shapiro S, Feldmesser M, Casadevall A, Scharff MD. 2001. Both Th1 and Th2 cytokines affect the ability of monoclonal antibodies to protect mice against *Cryptococcus neoformans*. Infect Immun 69:6445-6455.

Bellocchio S, Montagnoli C, Bozza S, Gaziano R, Rossi G, Mambula SS, Vecchi A, Mantovani A, Levitz SM, Romani L. 2004. The contribution of the Toll-like/IL-1 receptor superfamily to innate and adaptive immunity to fungal pathogens in vivo. J Immunol 172:3059-3069.

Bhatia S, Fei M, Yarlagadda M, Qi Z, Akira S, Saijo S, Iwakura Y, van Rooijen N, Gibson GA, St Croix CM, Ray A, Ray P. 2011. Rapid host defense against *Aspergillus fumigatus* involves alveolar macrophages with a predominance of alternatively activated phenotype. PLoS ONE 6:e15943.

Blackstock R, Buchanan KL, Adekunle M, Adesina, Murphy JW. 1999. Differential Regulation of Immune Responses by Highly and Weakly Virulent *Cryptococcus neoformans* Isolates. Infect Immun 67:3601-3609.

Blease K, Mehrad B, Standiford TJ, Lukacs NW, Gosling J, Boring L, Charo IF, Kunkel SL, Hogaboam CM. 2000. Enhanced pulmonary allergic responses to *Aspergillus* in CCR2-/- mice. J Immunol 165:2603-2611.

Bochud PY, Chien JW, Marr KA, Leisenring WM, Upton A, Janer M, Rodrigues SD, Li S, Hansen JA, Zhao LP, Aderem A, Boeckh M. 2008. Toll-like receptor 4 polymorphisms and aspergillosis in stem-cell transplantation. New Eng J Med 359:1766-1777.

Bonfim CV, Mamoni RL, Lima Blotta MHS. 2009. TLR-2, TLR-4 and dectin-1 expression in human monocytes and neutrophils stimulated by *Paracoccidioides brasiliensis*. Med Mycol 47:722-733.

Borger P, Koeter GH, Timmerman JA, Vellenga E, Tomee JF, Kauffman HF. 1999. Proteases from *Aspergillus fumigatus* induce interleukin (IL)-6 and IL-8 production in airway epithelial cell lines by transcriptional mechanisms. J Infect Dis 180:1267-1274.

Botterel F, Gross K, Ibrahim-Granet O, Khoufache K, Escabasse V, Coste A, Cordonnier C, Escudier E, Bretagne S. 2008. Phagocytosis of *Aspergillus fumigatus* conidia by primary nasal epithelial cells in vitro. BMC Microbiol 8:97.

Bozza S, Clavaud C, Giovannini G, Fontaine T, Beauvais A, Sarfati J, D'Angelo C, Perruccio K, Bonifazi P, Zagarella S, Moretti S, Bistoni F, Latge JP, Romani L. 2009. Immune sensing of *Aspergillus fumigatus* proteins, glycolipids, and polysaccharides and the impact on Th immunity and vaccination. J Immunol 183:2407-2414.

Bozza S, Gaziano R, Spreca A, Bacci A, Montagnoli C, di Francesco P, Romani L. 2002. Dendritic cells transport conidia and hyphae of *Aspergillus fumigatus* from the airways to the draining lymph nodes and initiate disparate Th responses to the fungus. J Immunol 168:1362-1371.

Bradsher RW, Balk RA, Jacobs RF. 1987. Growth inhibition of *Blastomyces dermatitidis* in alveolar and peripheral macrophages from patients with blastomycosis. Am Rev Resp Dis 135:412-417.

Brummer E, Castaneda E, Restrepo A. 1993. Paracoccidioidomycosis: an update. Clin Microbiol Rev 6:89-117.

Brummer E, Hanson LH, Restrepo A, Stevens DA. 1988. In vivo and in vitro activation of pulmonary macrophages by IFN-gamma for enhanced killing of *Paracoccidioides brasiliensis* or *Blastomyces dermatitidis*. J Immunol 140:2786-2789.

Brummer E, Kethineni N, Stevens DA. 2005. Immunological basis for susceptibility and resistance to pulmonary blastomycosis in mouse strains. Cytokine 32:12-19.

Brummer E, Kurita N, Yosihida S, Nishimura K, Miyaji M. 1991. Fungistatic activity of human neutrophils against *Histoplasma capsulatum*: correlation with phagocytosis. J Infect Dis 164:158-162.

Brummer E, Stevens DA. 1987. Fungicidal mechanisms of activated macrophages: evidence for nonoxidative mechanisms for killing of *Blastomyces dermatitidis*. Infect Immun 55:3221-3224.

Brummer E, Vinoda V, Stevens DA. 2006. IL-12 induction of resistance to pulmonary blastomycosis. Cytokine 35:221-228.

Bruns S, Kniemeyer O, Hasenberg M, Aimanianda V, Nietzsche S, Thywissen A, Jeron A, Latge JP, Brakhage AA, Gunzer M. 2010. Production of extracellular traps against *Aspergillus fumigatus* in vitro and in infected lung tissue is dependent on invading neutrophils and influenced by hydrophobin RodA. PLoS Pathog 6:e1000873.

Bryan RA, Jiang Z, Howell RC, Morgenstern A, Bruchertseifer F, Casadevall A, Dadachova E. 2010. Radioimmunotherapy is more effective than antifungal treatment in experimental cryptococcal infection. J Infect Dis 202:633-637.

Bullock WE, Wright SD. 1987. Role of the adherence-promoting receptors, CR3, LFA-1, and p150,95, in binding of *Histoplasma capsulatum* by human macrophages. J Exp Med 165:195-210.

Calderon EJ, Regordan C, Medrano FJ, Ollero M, Varela JM. 1996. *Pneumocystis carinii* infection in patients with chronic bronchial disease. Lancet 347:977.

Cano LE, Gomez B, Brummer E, Restrepo A, Stevens DA. 1994. Inhibitory effect of deferoxamine or macrophage activation on transformation of *Paracoccidioides brasiliensis* conidia ingested by macrophages: reversal by holotransferrin. Infect Immun 62:1494-1496.

Cano LE, Kashino SS, Arruda C, Andre D, Xidieh CF, Singer-Vermes LM, Vaz CA, Burger E, Calich VL. 1998. Protective role of gamma interferon in experimental pulmonary paracoccidioidomycosis. Infect Immun 66:800-806.

Cano LE, Singer-Vermes LM, Costa TA, Mengel JO, Xidieh CF, Arruda C, Andre DC, Vaz CA, Burger E, Calich VL. 2000. Depletion of CD8(+) T cells in vivo impairs host defense of mice resistant and susceptible to pulmonary paracoccidioidomycosis. Infect Immun 68:352-359.

Cano LE, Singer-Vermes LM, Vaz CA, Russo M, Calich VL. 1995. Pulmonary paracoccidioidomycosis in resistant and susceptible mice: relationship among progression of infection, bronchoalveolar cell activation, cellular immune response, and specific isotype patterns. Infect Immun 63:1777-1783.

Carmona EM, Lamont JD, Xue A, Wylam M, Limper AH. 2010. *Pneumocystis* cell wall beta-glucan stimulates calcium-dependent signaling of IL-8 secretion by human airway epithelial cells. Resp Res 11:95.

Carmona EM, Vassallo R, Vuk-Pavlovic Z, Standing JE, Kottom TJ, Limper AH. 2006. *Pneumocystis* cell wall beta-glucans induce dendritic cell costimulatory molecule expression and inflammatory activation through a Fas-Fas ligand mechanism. J Immunol 177:459-467.

Casadevall A, Cleare W, Feldmesser M, Glatman-Freedman A, Goldman DL, Kozel TR, Lendvai N, Mukherjee J, Pirofski LA, Rivera J, Rosas AL, Scharff MD, Valadon P,

Westin K, Zhong Z. 1998. Characterization of a murine monoclonal antibody to *Cryptococcus neoformans* polysaccharide that is a candidate for human therapeutic studies. Antimicrob Agents Chemother 42:1437-1446.

Casadevall A, Mukherjee J, Devi SJ, Schneerson R, Robbins JB, Scharff MD. 1992. Antibodies elicited by a *Cryptococcus neoformans*-tetanus toxoid conjugate vaccine have the same specificity as those elicited in infection. J Infect Dis 165:1086-1093.

Casadevall A, Pirofski LA. 2007. Antibody-mediated protection through cross-reactivity introduces a fungal heresy into immunological dogma. Infect Immun 75:5074-5078.

Cenci E, Mencacci A, Del Sero G, Bacci A, Montagnoli C, d'Ostiani CF, Mosci P, Bachmann M, Bistoni F, Kopf M, Romani L. 1999. Interleukin-4 causes susceptibility to invasive pulmonary aspergillosis through suppression of protective type I responses. J Infect Dis 180:1957-1968.

Cenci E, Perito S, Enssle KH, Mosci P, Latge JP, Romani L, Bistoni F. 1997. Th1 and Th2 cytokines in mice with invasive aspergillosis. Infect Immun 65:564-570.

Chamilos G, Ganguly D, Lande R, Gregorio J, Meller S, Goldman WE, Gilliet M, Kontoyiannis DP. 2010. Generation of IL-23 producing dendritic cells (DCs) by airborne fungi regulates fungal pathogenicity via the induction of T(H)-17 responses. PLoS ONE 5:e12955.

Chen GH, McNamara DA, Hernandez Y, Huffnagle GB, Toews GB, Olszewski MA. 2008. Inheritance of Immune Polarization Patterns Is Linked to Resistance versus Susceptibility to *Cryptococcus neoformans* in a Mouse Model. Infect Immun 76:2379-2391.

Chen GH, Olszewski MA, McDonald RA, Wells JC, Paine R, 3rd, Huffnagle GB, Toews GB. 2007. Role of granulocyte macrophage colony-stimulating factor in host defense against pulmonary *Cryptococcus neoformans* infection during murine allergic bronchopulmonary mycosis. Am J Pathol 170:1028-1040.

Cheng BH, Liu Y, Xuei X, Liao CP, Lu D, Lasbury ME, Durant PJ, Lee CH. 2010. Microarray studies on effects of *Pneumocystis carinii* infection on global gene expression in alveolar macrophages. BMC Microbiol 10:103.

Cher DJ, Mosmann TR. 1987. Two types of murine helper T cell clone. II. Delayed-type hypersensitivity is mediated by TH1 clones. J Immunol 138:3688-3694.

Cherwinski HM, Schumacher JH, Brown KD, Mosmann TR. 1987. Two types of mouse helper T cell clone. III. Further differences in lymphokine synthesis between Th1 and Th2 clones revealed by RNA hybridization, functionally monospecific bioassays, and monoclonal antibodies. J Exp Med 166:1229-1244.

Chuck SL, Sande MA. 1989. Infections with *Cryptococcus neoformans* in the Acquired Immunodeficiency Syndrome. New Engl J Med 321:794-799.

Cole GT, Xue JM, Okeke CN, Tarcha EJ, Basrur V, Schaller RA, Herr RA, Yu JJ, Hung CY. 2004. A vaccine against coccidioidomycosis is justified and attainable. Med Mycol 42:189-216.

Conti HR, Shen F, Nayyar N, Stocum E, Sun JN, Lindemann MJ, Ho AW, Hai JH, Yu JJ, Jung JW, Filler SG, Masso-Welch P, Edgerton M, Gaffen SL. 2009. Th17 cells and IL-17 receptor signaling are essential for mucosal host defense against oral candidiasis. J Exp Med 206:299-311.

Cox RA, Magee DM. 2004. Coccidioidomycosis: host response and vaccine development. Clin Microbiol Rev 17:804-839

Cutler JE, Deepe GS, Jr., Klein BS. 2007. Advances in combating fungal diseases: vaccines on the threshold. Nat Rev Microbiol 5:13-28.

D'Angelo C, De Luca A, Zelante T, Bonifazi P, Moretti S, Giovannini G, Iannitti RG, Zagarella S, Bozza S, Campo S, Salvatori G, Romani L. 2009. Exogenous pentraxin 3 restores antifungal resistance and restrains inflammation in murine chronic granulomatous disease. J Immunol 183:4609-4618.

Dadachova E, Nakouzi A, Bryan RA, Casadevall A. 2003. Ionizing radiation delivered by specific antibody is therapeutic against a fungal infection. Proc Natl Acad Sci U S A 100:10942-10947.

Dan JM, Wang JP, Lee CK, Levitz SM. 2008. Cooperative Stimulation of Dendritic Cells by *Cryptococcus neoformans* Mannoproteins and CpG Oligodeoxynucleotides. PLoS ONE 3:e2046.

Datta K, Lees A, Pirofski LA. 2008. Therapeutic efficacy of a conjugate vaccine containing a peptide mimotope of cryptococcal capsular polysaccharide glucuronoxylomannan. Clin Vaccine Immunol 15:1176-1187.

Davis JL, Welsh DA, Beard CB, Jones JL, Lawrence GG, Fox MR, Crothers K, Morris A, Charbonnet D, Swartzman A, Huang L. 2008. *Pneumocystis* colonisation is common among hospitalised HIV infected patients with non-*Pneumocystis* pneumonia. Thorax 63:329-334.

de Bastos Ascenco Soares R, Gomez FJ, de Almeida Soares CM, Deepe GS, Jr. 2008. Vaccination with heat shock protein 60 induces a protective immune response against experimental *Paracoccidioides brasiliensis* pulmonary infection. Infect Immun 76:4214-4221.

de Luca A, Bozza S, Zelante T, Zagarella S, D'Angelo C, Perruccio K, Vacca C, Carvalho A, Cunha C, Aversa F, Romani L. 2010a. Non-hematopoietic cells contribute to protective tolerance to *Aspergillus fumigatus* via a TRIF pathway converging on IDO. Cell Mol Immunol 7:459-470.

De Luca A, Zelante T, D'Angelo C, Zagarella S, Fallarino F, Spreca A, Iannitti RG, Bonifazi P, Renauld JC, Bistoni F, Puccetti P, Romani L. 2010b. IL-22 defines a novel immune pathway of antifungal resistance. Mucosal Immunol 3:361-373.

Deacon L, Pankhurst L, Liu J, Drew GH, Hayes ET, Jackson S, Longhurst J, Longhurst P, Pollard S, Tyrrel S. 2009. Endotoxin emissions from commercial composting activities. Environ Health 8 Suppl 1:S9.

Deepe G. 2005. The Innate and Adaptive Immune Response to Pulmonary *Histoplasma capsulatum* Infection. In: Fidel P, Huffnagle G, editors. Fungal Immunology: Springer US. p 85-112.

Deepe GS, Jr. 2000. Immune response to early and late *Histoplasma capsulatum* infections. Curr Opin Microbiol 3:359-362.

Deepe GS, Jr., Gibbons RS. 2002. Cellular and molecular regulation of vaccination with heat shock protein 60 from *Histoplasma capsulatum*. Infect Immun 70:3759-3767.

Deepe GS, Jr., Gibbons RS. 2006. T cells require tumor necrosis factor-alpha to provide protective immunity in mice infected with *Histoplasma capsulatum*. J Infect Dis 193:322-330.

Deepe GS, Jr., Watson SR, Bullock WE. 1984. Cellular origins and target cells of immunoregulatory factors in mice with disseminated histoplasmosis. J Immunol 132:2064-2071.

Del Poeta M. 2004. Role of Phagocytosis in the Virulence of *Cryptococcus neoformans*. Eukaryotic Cell 3:1067-1075.

Denning DW. 1996. Aspergillosis: diagnosis and treatment. Int J Antimicrob Agents 6:161-168.

Devi SJ. 1996. Preclinical efficacy of a glucuronoxylomannan-tetanus toxoid conjugate vaccine of *Cryptococcus neoformans* in a murine model. Vaccine 14:841-844.

Devi SJ, Schneerson R, Egan W, Ulrich TJ, Bryla D, Robbins JB, Bennett JE. 1991. *Cryptococcus neoformans* serotype A glucuronoxylomannan-protein conjugate vaccines: synthesis, characterization, and immunogenicity. Infect Immun 59:3700-3707.

Dias MF, Mesquita J, Filgueira AL, De Souza W. 2008. Human neutrophils susceptibility to *Paracoccidioides brasiliensis*: an ultrastructural and cytochemical assay. Med Mycology 46:241-249.

Diaz-Arevalo D, Bagramyan K, Hong TB, Ito JI, Kalkum M. 2011. CD4(+) T cells mediate the protective effect of the recombinant Asp f3-based anti-aspergillosis vaccine. Infect Immun 79:2257-2266.

Dionne SO, Podany AB, Ruiz YW, Ampel NM, Galgiani JN, Lake DF. 2006. Spherules derived from *Coccidioides posadasii* promote human dendritic cell maturation and activation. Infect Immun 74:2415-2422.

Drutz DJ, Frey CL. 1985. Intracellular and extracellular defenses of human phagocytes against *Blastomyces dermatitidis* conidia and yeasts. J Lab Clin Med 105:737-750.

Drutz DJ, Huppert M. 1983. Coccidioidomycosis: factors affecting the host-parasite interaction. Journal Infect Dis 147:372-390.

Eissenberg LG, Goldman WE. 1988. Fusion of lysosomes with phagosomes containing *Histoplasma capsulatum*: use of fluoresceinated dextran. Adv Exp Med Biol 239:53-61.

Eissenberg LG, Goldman WE, Schlesinger PH. 1993. *Histoplasma capsulatum* modulates the acidification of phagolysosomes. J Exp Med 177:1605-1611.

Eissenberg LG, Schlesinger PH, Goldman WE. 1988. Phagosome-lysosome fusion in P388D1 macrophages infected with *Histoplasma capsulatum*. J Leuk Biol 43:483-491.

Ersland K, Wuthrich M, Klein BS. 2010. Dynamic interplay among monocyte-derived, dermal, and resident lymph node dendritic cells during the generation of vaccine immunity to fungi. Cell Host Microbe 7:474-487.

Evans SE, Hahn PY, McCann F, Kottom TJ, Pavlovic ZV, Limper AH. 2005. Pneumocystis cell wall beta-glucans stimulate alveolar epithelial cell chemokine generation through nuclear factor-kappaB-dependent mechanisms. Am J Resp Cell Mol Biol 32:490-497.

Eyerich S, Eyerich K, Pennino D, Carbone T, Nasorri F, Pallotta S, Cianfarani F, Odorisio T, Traidl-Hoffmann C, Behrendt H, Durham SR, Schmidt-Weber CB, Cavani A. 2009. Th22 cells represent a distinct human T cell subset involved in epidermal immunity and remodeling. J Clin Invest 119:3573-3585.

Ezekowitz RA, Williams DJ, Koziel H, Armstrong MY, Warner A, Richards FF, Rose RM. 1991. Uptake of *Pneumocystis carinii* mediated by the macrophage mannose receptor. Nature 351:155-158.

Fernandez-Botran R, Sanders VM, Mosmann TR, Vitetta ES. 1988. Lymphokine-mediated regulation of the proliferative response of clones of T helper 1 and T helper 2 cells. J Exp Med 168:543-558.

Ferreira KS, Lopes JD, Almeida SR. 2004. Down-regulation of dendritic cell activation induced by *Paracoccidioides brasiliensis*. Immunol Lett 94:107-114.

Fierer J, Waters C, Walls L. 2006. Both CD4+ and CD8+ T cells can mediate vaccine-induced protection against *Coccidioides immitis* infection in mice. J Infect Dis 193:1323-1331.

Fisher FS, Bultman MW, Johnson SM, Pappagianis D, Zaborsky E. 2007. *Coccidioides* niches and habitat parameters in the southwestern United States: a matter of scale. Ann N Y Acad Sci 1111:47-72.

Fleuridor R, Lees A, Pirofski L. 2001. A cryptococcal capsular polysaccharide mimotope prolongs the survival of mice with *Cryptococcus neoformans* infection. J Immunol 166:1087-1096.

Fleuridor R, Zhong Z, Pirofski L. 1998. A human IgM monoclonal antibody prolongs survival of mice with lethal cryptococcosis. J Infect Dis 178:1213-1216.

Fleury J, Escudier E, Pocholle MJ, Carre C, Bernaudin JF. 1985. Cell population obtained by bronchoalveolar lavage in *Pneumocystis carinii* pneumonitis. Acta Cytol 29:721-726.

Franco M. 1987. Host-parasite relationships in paracoccidioidomycosis. J Med Vet Mycol 25:5-18.

Franco M, Sano A, Kera K, Nishimura K, Takeo K, Miyaji M. 1989. Chlamydospore formation by *Paracoccidioides brasiliensis* mycelial form. Rev Inst Med Trop Sao Paulo 31:151-157.

Fraser IP, Takahashi K, Koziel H, Fardin B, Harmsen A, Ezekowitz RA. 2000. *Pneumocystis carinii* enhances soluble mannose receptor production by macrophages. Microbes Infect 2:1305-1310.

Frey CL, Drutz DJ. 1986. Influence of fungal surface components on the interaction of *Coccidioides immitis* with polymorphonuclear neutrophils. The Journal of Infectious Diseases 153:933-943.

Frosco MB, Chase T, Jr., Macmillan JD. 1994. The effect of elastase-specific monoclonal and polyclonal antibodies on the virulence of *Aspergillus fumigatus* in immunocompromised mice. Mycopathologia 125:65-76.

Fujita H, Nograles KE, Kikuchi T, Gonzalez J, Carucci JA, Krueger JG. 2009. Human Langerhans cells induce distinct IL-22-producing CD4+ T cells lacking IL-17 production. Proc Natl Acad Sci U S A 106:21795-21800.

Gafa V, Remoli ME, Giacomini E, Gagliardi MC, Lande R, Severa M, Grillot R, Coccia EM. 2007. In vitro infection of human dendritic cells by *Aspergillus fumigatus* conidia triggers the secretion of chemokines for neutrophil and Th1 lymphocyte recruitment. Microbes Infect 9:971-980.

Gajewski TF, Fitch FW. 1988. Anti-proliferative effect of IFN-gamma in immune regulation. I. IFN-gamma inhibits the proliferation of Th2 but not Th1 murine helper T lymphocyte clones. J Immunol 140:4245-4252.

Galgiani JN. 1986. Inhibition of Different Phases of *Coccidioides immitis* by Human Neutrophils or Hydrogen Peroxide. Journal of Infectious Diseases 153:217-222.

Gereke M, Jung S, Buer J, Bruder D. 2009. Alveolar type II epithelial cells present antigen to CD4(+) T cells and induce Foxp3(+) regulatory T cells. Am J Respir Crit Care Med 179:344-355.

Gersuk GM, Underhill DM, Zhu L, Marr KA. 2006. Dectin-1 and TLRs permit macrophages to distinguish between different *Aspergillus fumigatus* cellular states. J Immunol 176:3717-3724.

Gigliotti F, Haidaris CG, Wright TW, Harmsen AG. 2002. Passive intranasal monoclonal antibody prophylaxis against murine *Pneumocystis carinii* pneumonia. Infect Immun 70:1069-1074.

Gigliotti F, Hughes WT. 1988. Passive immunoprophylaxis with specific monoclonal antibody confers partial protection against *Pneumocystis carinii* pneumonitis in animal models. J Clin Invest 81:1666-1668.

Gildea LA, Ciraolo GM, Morris RE, Newman SL. 2005. Human dendritic cell activity against *Histoplasma capsulatum* is mediated via phagolysosomal fusion. Infect Immun 73:6803-6811.

Gildea LA, Morris RE, Newman SL. 2001. *Histoplasma capsulatum* yeasts are phagocytosed via very late antigen-5, killed, and processed for antigen presentation by human dendritic cells. J Immunol 166:1049-1056.

Goihman-Yahr M, Essenfeld-Yahr E, de Albornoz MC, Yarzabal L, de Gomez MH, San Martin B, Ocanto A, Gil F, Convit J. 1980. Defect of in vitro digestive ability of polymorphonuclear leukocytes in paracoccidioidomycosis. Infect Immun 28:557-566.

Goihman-Yahr M, Pereira J, Isturiz G, Viloria N, Carrasquero M, Saavedra N, de Gomez MH, Roman A, San Martin B, Bastardo de Albornoz MC, et al. 1992. Relationship between digestive and killing abilities of neutrophils against *Paracoccidioides brasiliensis*. Mycoses 35:269-274.

Goihman-Yahr M, Rothenberg A, Rosquete R, Avila-Millan E, de Albornoz MC, de Gomez MH, San Martin B, Ocanto A, Pereira J, Molina T. 1985. A novel method for estimating killing ability and digestion of *Paracoccidioides brasiliensis* by phagocytic cells in vitro. Sabouraudia 23:245-251.

Gomez FJ, Allendoerfer R, Deepe GS, Jr. 1995. Vaccination with recombinant heat shock protein 60 from *Histoplasma capsulatum* protects mice against pulmonary histoplasmosis. Infect Immun 63:2587-2595.

Gomez FJ, Pilcher-Roberts R, Alborzi A, Newman SL. 2008. *Histoplasma capsulatum* cyclophilin A mediates attachment to dendritic cell VLA-5. J Immunol 181:7106-7114.

Gomez P, Hackett TL, Moore MM, Knight DA, Tebbutt SJ. 2010. Functional genomics of human bronchial epithelial cells directly interacting with conidia of *Aspergillus fumigatus*. BMC Genomics 11:358.

Gonzalez A, de Gregori W, Velez D, Restrepo A, Cano LE. 2000. Nitric Oxide Participation in the Fungicidal Mechanism of Gamma Interferon-Activated Murine Macrophages against *Paracoccidioides brasiliensis* Conidia. Infect Immun 68:2546-2552.

Granger DL, Hibbs JB, Jr., Perfect JR, Durack DT. 1990. Metabolic fate of L-arginine in relation to microbiostatic capability of murine macrophages. J Clin Invest 85:264-273.

Grazziutti M, Przepiorka D, Rex JH, Braunschweig I, Vadhan-Raj S, Savary CA. 2001. Dendritic cell-mediated stimulation of the in vitro lymphocyte response to *Aspergillus*. Bone Marrow Transplant 27:647-652.

Guerrero A, Jain N, Wang X, Fries BC. 2010. *Cryptococcus neoformans* variants generated by phenotypic switching differ in virulence through effects on macrophage activation. Infect Immun 78:1049-1057.

Guillot L, Carroll SF, Badawy M, Qureshi ST. 2008a. *Cryptococcus neoformans* induces IL-8 secretion and CXCL1 expression by human bronchial epithelial cells. Resp Res 9:9.

Guillot L, Carroll SF, Homer R, Qureshi ST. 2008b. Enhanced innate immune responsiveness to pulmonary *Cryptococcus neoformans* infection is associated with resistance to progressive infection. Infect Immun 76:4745-4756.

Hanano R, Kaufmann SH. 1999. *Pneumocystis carinii* pneumonia in mutant mice deficient in both TCRalphabeta and TCRgammadelta cells: cytokine and antibody responses. J Infect Dis 179:455-459.

Hanna SA, Monteiro da Silva JL, Giannini MJ. 2000. Adherence and intracellular parasitism of *Paracoccidioides brasiliensis* in Vero cells. Microbes Infect 2:877-884.

Hardison SE, Ravi S, Wozniak KL, Young ML, Olszewski MA, Wormley FL, Jr. 2010a. Pulmonary Infection with an Interferon-{gamma}-Producing *Cryptococcus neoformans* Strain Results in Classical Macrophage Activation and Protection. Am J Pathol 176:774-785.

Hardison SE, Wozniak KL, Kolls JK, Wormley FL, Jr. 2010b. Interleukin-17 Is Not Required for Classical Macrophage Activation in a Pulmonary Mouse Model of *Cryptococcus neoformans* Infection. Infect Immun 78:5341-5351.

Harmsen AG, Stankiewicz M. 1990. Requirement for CD4+ cells in resistance to *Pneumocystis carinii* pneumonia in mice. J Exp Med 172:937-945.

Harmsen AG, Stankiewicz M. 1991. T cells are not sufficient for resistance to *Pneumocystis carinii* pneumonia in mice. J Protozool 38:44S-45S.

Hasenberg M, A KH, Bonifatius S, Jeron A, Gunzer M. 2011. Direct Observation of Phagocytosis and NET-formation by Neutrophils in Infected Lungs using 2-photon Microscopy. J Vis Exp.

Hernandez Y, Arora S, Erb-Downward JR, McDonald RA, Toews GB, Huffnagle GB. 2005. Distinct roles for IL-4 and IL-10 in regulating T2 immunity during allergic bronchopulmonary mycosis. J Immunol 174:1027-1036.

Herring AC, Falkowski NR, Chen GH, McDonald RA, Toews GB, Huffnagle GB. 2005. Transient neutralization of tumor necrosis factor alpha can produce a chronic fungal infection in an immunocompetent host: Potential role of immature dendritic cells. Infect Immun 73:39-49.

Herring AC, Lee J, McDonald RA, Toews GB, Huffnagle GB. 2002. Induction of interleukin-12 and gamma interferon requires tumor necrosis factor alpha for protective T1-cell-mediated immunity to pulmonary *Cryptococcus neoformans* infection. Infect Immun 70:2959-2964.

Hidore MR, Mislan TW, Murphy JW. 1991a. Responses of murine natural killer cells to binding of the fungal target *Cryptococcus neoformans*. Infect Immun 59:1489-1499.

Hidore MR, Murphy JW. 1989. Murine natural killer cell interactions with a fungal target, *Cryptococcus neoformans*. Infect Immun 57:1990-1997.

Hidore MR, Nabavi N, Sonleitner F, Murphy JW. 1991b. Murine natural killer cells are fungicidal to Cryptococcus neoformans. Infection and immunity 59:1747-1754.

Hu T, Takamoto M, Hida S, Tagawa Y, Sugane K. 2009. IFN-gamma deficiency worsen Pneumocystis pneumonia with Th17 development in nude mice. Immunol Lett 127:55-59.

Huang L, Crothers K, Morris A, Groner G, Fox M, Turner JR, Merrifield C, Eiser S, Zucchi P, Beard CB. 2003. Pneumocystis colonization in HIV-infected patients. J Eukaryot Microbiol 50 Suppl:616-617.

Huffnagle GB, Lipscomb MF. 1992. Pulmonary cryptococcosis. Am J Pathol 141:1517-1520.

Huffnagle GB, Lipscomb MF, Lovchik JA, Hoag KA, Street NE. 1994. The role of CD4(+) and CD8(+) T-Cells in the protective inflammatory response to a pulmonary cryptococcal infection. J Leukoc Biol 55:35-42.

Huffnagle GB, Yates JL, Lipscomb MF. 1991. T-cell-mediated immunity in the lung - a *Cryptococcus neoformans* pulmonary infection model using SCID and athymic nude-mice. Infect Immun 59:1423-1433.

Ibrahim-Granet O, Philippe B, Boleti H, Boisvieux-Ulrich E, Grenet D, Stern M, Latge JP. 2003. Phagocytosis and Intracellular Fate of *Aspergillus fumigatus* Conidia in Alveolar Macrophages. Infect Immun 71:891-903.

Jain AV, Zhang Y, Fields WB, McNamara DA, Choe MY, Chen GH, Erb-Downward J, Osterholzer JJ, Toews GB, Huffnagle GB, Olszewski MA. 2009. Th2 but not Th1 immune bias results in altered lung functions in a murine model of pulmonary *Cryptococcus neoformans* infection. Infect Immun 77:5389-5399.

Jarvis JN, Harrison TS. 2007. HIV-associated cryptococcal meningitis. AIDS 21:2119-2129.

Jimenez BE, Murphy JW. 1984. In vitro effects of natural killer cells against *Paracoccidioides brasiliensis* yeast phase. Infect Immun 46:552-558.

Johnston SA, May RC. 2010. The human fungal pathogen *Cryptococcus neoformans* escapes macrophages by a phagosome emptying mechanism that is inhibited by Arp2/3 complex-mediated actin polymerisation. PLoS Pathog 6.

Kagi MK, Fierz W, Grob PJ, Russi EW. 1993. High proportion of gamma-delta T cell receptor positive T cells in bronchoalveolar lavage and peripheral blood of HIV-infected patients with *Pneumocystis carinii* pneumonias. Respiration 60:170-177.

Kappe R, Levitz S, Harrison TS, Ruhnke M, Ampel NM, Just-Nubling G. 1998. Recent advances in cryptococcosis, candidiasis and coccidioidomycosis complicating HIV infection. Med Mycol 36:207-215.

Kashkin KP, Likholetov SM, Lipnitsky AV. 1977. Studies on mediators of cellular immunity in experimental coccidioidomycosis. Sabouraudia 15:59-68.

Kasperkovitz PV, Cardenas ML, Vyas JM. 2010. TLR9 is actively recruited to *Aspergillus fumigatus* phagosomes and requires the N-terminal proteolytic cleavage domain for proper intracellular trafficking. J Immunol 185:7614-7622.

Kawakami K, Kinjo Y, Uezu K, Yara S, Miyagi K, Koguchi Y, Nakayama T, Taniguchi M, Saito A. 2001a. Monocyte chemoattractant protein-1-dependent increase of V alpha 14 NKT cells in lungs and their roles in Th1 response and host defense in cryptococcal infection. J Immunol 167:6525-6532.

Kawakami K, Kinjo Y, Yara S, Koguchi Y, Uezu K, Nakayama T, Taniguchi M, Saito A. 2001b. Activation of Valpha14(+) natural killer T cells by alpha-galactosylceramide results in development of Th1 response and local host resistance in mice infected with *Cryptococcus neoformans*. Infect Immun 69:213-220.

Kawakami K, Kinjo Y, Yara S, Uezu K, Koguchi Y, Tohyama M, Azuma M, Takeda K, Akira S, Saito A. 2001c. Enhanced gamma interferon production through activation of Valpha14(+) natural killer T cells by alpha-galactosylceramide in interleukin-18-deficient mice with systemic cryptococcosis. Infect Immun 69:6643-6650.

Kawakami K, Qureshi MH, Zhang T, Okamura H, Kurimoto M, Saito A. 1997. IL-18 protects mice against pulmonary and disseminated infection with *Cryptococcus neoformans* by inducing IFN-gamma production. J Immunol 159:5528-5534.

Kawakami K, Shibuya K, Qureshi MH, Zhang TT, Koguchi Y, Tohyama M, Xie QF, Naoe S, Saito A. 1999. Chemokine responses and accumulation of inflammatory cells in the lungs of mice infected with highly virulent *Cryptococcus neoformans*: effects of interleukin-12. FEMS Immunol Med Microbiol 25:391-402.

Keely SP, Stringer JR, Baughman RP, Linke MJ, Walzer PD, Smulian AG. 1995. Genetic variation among *Pneumocystis carinii* hominis isolates in recurrent pneumocystosis. J Infect Dis 172:595-598.

Kelly MN, Shellito JE. 2010. Current understanding of *Pneumocystis* immunology. Future Microbiol 5:43-65.

Kelly RM, Chen JM, Yauch LE, Levitz SM. 2005. Opsonic requirements for dendritic cell-mediated responses to *Cryptococcus neoformans*. Infect Immun 73:592-598.

Kethineni N, Brummer E, Stevens DA. 2006. Susceptibility to pulmonary blastomycosis in young compared to adult mice: immune deficiencies in young mice. Med Mycol 44:51-60.

Kimberlin CL, Hariri AR, Hempel HO, Goodman NL. 1981. Interactions between Histoplasma capsulatum and macrophages from normal and treated mice: comparison of the mycelial and yeast phases in alveolar and peritoneal macrophages. Infect Immun 34:6-10.

Klein BS, Hogan LH, Jones JM. 1993. Immunologic recognition of a 25-amino acid repeat arrayed in tandem on a major antigen of *Blastomyces dermatitidis*. J Clin Invest 92:330-337.

Klein BS, Vergeront JM, Weeks RJ, Kumar UN, Mathai G, Varkey B, Kaufman L, Bradsher RW, Stoebig JF, Davis JP. 1986. Isolation of *Blastomyces dermatitidis* in soil associated with a large outbreak of blastomycosis in Wisconsin. New Engl J Med 314:529-534.

Kleinschek MA, Muller U, Schutze N, Sabat R, Straubinger RK, Blumenschein WM, McClanahan T, Kastelein RA, Alber G. 2010. Administration of IL-23 engages innate and adaptive immune mechanisms during fungal infection. Int Immunol 22:81-90.

Kling HM, Shipley TW, Patil S, Morris A, Norris KA. 2009. *Pneumocystis* colonization in immunocompetent and simian immunodeficiency virus-infected cynomolgus macaques. J Infect Dis 199:89-96.

Kobayashi H, Worgall S, O'Connor TP, Crystal RG. 2007. Interaction of *Pneumocystis carinii* with dendritic cells and resulting host responses to *P. carinii*. J Immunother (1997) 30:54-63.

Kong YM, Savage DC, Levine HB. 1965. Enhancement of immune responses in mice by a booster injection of *Coccidioides* spherules. J Immunol 95:1048-1056.

Kontoyiannis DP. 2010. Manipulation of host angioneogenesis: A critical link for understanding the pathogenesis of invasive mold infections? Virulence 1:192-196.

Kovacs JA, Kovacs AA, Polis M, Wright WC, Gill VJ, Tuazon CU, Gelmann EP, Lane HC, Longfield R, Overturf G, Macher AM, Fauci AS, Parrillo JE, Bennett JE, Masur H. 1985. Cryptococcosis in the Acquired Immunodeficiency Syndrome. Ann Intern Med 103:533-538.

Kozel TR, Pfrommer GS, Redelman D. 1987. Activated neutrophils exhibit enhanced phagocytosis of *Cryptococcus neoformans* opsonized with normal human serum. Clin Exp Immunol 70:238-246.

Koziel H, Eichbaum Q, Kruskal BA, Pinkston P, Rogers RA, Armstrong MY, Richards FF, Rose RM, Ezekowitz RA. 1998. Reduced binding and phagocytosis of *Pneumocystis carinii* by alveolar macrophages from persons infected with HIV-1 correlates with mannose receptor downregulation. J Clin Invest 102:1332-1344.

Kroetz DN, Deepe GS, Jr. 2010. CCR5 dictates the equilibrium of proinflammatory IL-17+ and regulatory Foxp3+ T cells in fungal infection. J Immunol 184:5224-5231.

Kurita N, Brummer E, Yoshida S, Nishimura K, Miyaji M. 1991a. Antifungal activity of murine polymorphonuclear neutrophils against *Histoplasma capsulatum*. J Med Vet Mycol 29:133-143.

Kurita N, Terao K, Brummer E, Ito E, Nishimura K, Miyaji M. 1991b. Resistance of *Histoplasma capsulatum* to killing by human neutrophils. Evasion of oxidative burst and lysosomal-fusion products. Mycopathologia 115:207-213.

Lanken PN, Minda M, Pietra GG, Fishman AP. 1980. Alveolar response to experimental *Pneumocystis carinii* pneumonia in the rat. Am J Pathol 99:561-588.

Latge JP. 1999. *Aspergillus fumigatus* and aspergillosis. Clin Microbiol Rev 12:310-350.

Leigh TR, Millett MJ, Jameson B, Collins JV. 1993. Serum titres of *Pneumocystis carinii* antibody in health care workers caring for patients with AIDS. Thorax 48:619-621.

Levitz SM. 1991. The ecology of *Cryptococcus neoformans* and the epidemiology of cryptococcosis. Rev Infect Dis 13:1163-1169.

Levitz SM, Dupont MP. 1993. Phenotypic and functional characterization of human lymphocytes activated by interleukin-2 to directly inhibit growth of *Cryptococcus neoformans* in vitro. Journal Clin Invest 91:1490-1498.

Levitz SM, Nong SH, Seetoo KF, Harrison TS, Speizer RA, Simons ER. 1999. *Cryptococcus neoformans* resides in an acidic phagolysosome of human macrophages. Infect Immun 67:885-890.

Li K, Yu JJ, Hung CY, Lehmann PF, Cole GT. 2001. Recombinant urease and urease DNA of *Coccidioides immitis* elicit an immunoprotective response against coccidioidomycosis in mice. Infect Immun 69:2878-2887.

Lim TS, Murphy JW. 1980. Transfer of immunity to cryptococcosis by T-enriched splenic lymphocytes from *Cryptococcus neoformans*-sensitized mice. Infect Immun 30:5-11.

Lin JS, Huang JH, Hung LY, Wu SY, Wu-Hsieh BA. 2010. Distinct roles of complement receptor 3, Dectin-1, and sialic acids in murine macrophage interaction with *Histoplasma* yeast. J Leuk Biol 88:95-106.

Lindell DM, Moore TA, McDonald RA, Toews GB, Huffnagle GB. 2006. Distinct compartmentalization of CD4+ T-cell effector function versus proliferative capacity during pulmonary cryptococcosis. Am J Pathol 168:847-855.

Lipscomb MF, Alvarellos T, Toews GB, Tompkins R, Evans Z, Koo G, Kumar V. 1987. Role of natural killer cells in resistance to *Cryptococcus neoformans* infections in mice. Am J Pathol 128:354-361.

Littman DR, Rudensky AY. 2010. Th17 and regulatory T cells in mediating and restraining inflammation. Cell 140:845-858.

Long EG, Smith JS, Meier JL. 1986. Attachment of *Pneumocystis carinii* to rat pneumocytes. Laboratory investigation; a journal of technical methods and pathology 54:609-615.

Long KH, Gomez FJ, Morris RE, Newman SL. 2003. Identification of heat shock protein 60 as the ligand on *Histoplasma capsulatum* that mediates binding to CD18 receptors on human macrophages. J Immunol 170:487-494.

Loures FV, Pina A, Felonato M, Calich VL. 2009. TLR2 is a negative regulator of Th17 cells and tissue pathology in a pulmonary model of fungal infection. J Immunol 183:1279-1290.

Lund FE, Hollifield M, Schuer K, Lines JL, Randall TD, Garvy BA. 2006. B cells are required for generation of protective effector and memory CD4 cells in response to *Pneumocystis* lung infection. J Immunol 176:6147-6154.

Lund FE, Schuer K, Hollifield M, Randall TD, Garvy BA. 2003. Clearance of *Pneumocystis carinii* in mice is dependent on B cells but not on *P carinii*-specific antibody. J Immunol 171:1423-1430.

Ma H, Croudace JE, Lammas DA, May RC. 2006. Expulsion of live pathogenic yeast by macrophages. Curr Biol 16:2156-2160.

Ma LL, Spurrell JC, Wang JF, Neely GG, Epelman S, Krensky AM, Mody CH. 2002. CD8 T cell-mediated killing of *Cryptococcus neoformans* requires granulysin and is dependent on CD4 T cells and IL-15. J Immunol 169:5787-5795.

Ma LL, Wang CL, Neely GG, Epelman S, Krensky AM, Mody CH. 2004. NK cells use perforin rather than granulysin for anticryptococcal activity. J Immunol 173:3357-3365.

Magill SS, Chiller TM, Warnock DW. 2008. Evolving strategies in the management of aspergillosis. Expert Opin Pharmacother 9:193-209.

Maitta RW, Datta K, Chang Q, Luo RX, Witover B, Subramaniam K, Pirofski LA. 2004. Protective and nonprotective human immunoglobulin M monoclonal antibodies to *Cryptococcus neoformans* glucuronoxylomannan manifest different specificities and gene use profiles. Infect Immun 72:4810-4818.

Mambula SS, Sau K, Henneke P, Golenbock DT, Levitz SM. 2002. Toll-like receptor (TLR) signaling in response to *Aspergillus fumigatus*. J Biol Chem 277:39320-39326.

Mambula SS, Simons ER, Hastey R, Selsted ME, Levitz SM. 2000. Human neutrophil-mediated nonoxidative antifungal activity against *Cryptococcus neoformans*. Infect Immun 68:6257-6264.

Mansour MK, Latz E, Levitz SM. 2006. *Cryptococcus neoformans* glycoantigens are captured by multiple lectin receptors and presented by dendritic cells. J Immunol 176:3053-3061.

Mantovani A, Muzio M, Garlanda C, Sozzani S, Allavena P. 2001. Macrophage control of inflammation: negative pathways of regulation of inflammatory cytokines. Novartis Found Symp 234:120-131.

Marcotte H, Levesque D, Delanay K, Bourgeault A, de la Durantaye R, Brochu S, Lavoie MC. 1996. *Pneumocystis carinii* infection in transgenic B cell-deficient mice. J Infect Dis 173:1034-1037.

Marr KJ, Jones GJ, Zheng C, Huston SM, Timm-McCann M, Islam A, Berenger BM, Ma LL, Wiseman JC, Mody CH. 2009. *Cryptococcus neoformans* directly stimulates perforin production and rearms NK cells for enhanced anticryptococcal microbicidal activity. Infect Immun 77:2436-2446.

McKinley L, Logar AJ, McAllister F, Zheng M, Steele C, Kolls JK. 2006. Regulatory T cells dampen pulmonary inflammation and lung injury in an animal model of *Pneumocystis* pneumonia. J Immunol 177:6215-6226.

Mednick AJ, Feldmesser M, Rivera J, Casadevall A. 2003. Neutropenia alters lung cytokine production in mice and reduces their susceptibility to pulmonary cryptococcosis. Eur J Immunol 33:1744-1753.

Meier A, Kirschning CJ, Nikolaus T, Wagner H, Heesemann J, Ebel F. 2003. Toll-like receptor (TLR) 2 and TLR4 are essential for *Aspergillus*-induced activation of murine macrophages. Cell Microbiol 5:561-570.

Mendes-Giannini MJ, Hanna SA, da Silva JL, Andreotti PF, Vincenzi LR, Benard G, Lenzi HL, Soares CP. 2004. Invasion of epithelial mammalian cells by *Paracoccidioides brasiliensis* leads to cytoskeletal rearrangement and apoptosis of the host cell. Microbes Infect 6:882-891.

Mendes-Giannini MJ, Ricci LC, Uemura MA, Toscano E, Arns CW. 1994. Infection and apparent invasion of Vero cells by *Paracoccidioides brasiliensis*. J Med Vet Mycol 32:189-197.

Merkel GJ, Scofield BA. 1997. The in vitro interaction of *Cryptococcus neoformans* with human lung epithelial cells. FEMS Immunol Med Microbiol 19:203-213.

Millard PR, Wakefield AE, Hopkin JM. 1990. A sequential ultrastructural study of rat lungs infected with *Pneumocystis carinii* to investigate the appearances of the organism, its relationships and its effects on pneumocytes. Int J Exp Pathol 71:895-904.

Miller MF, Mitchell TG, Storkus WJ, Dawson JR. 1990. Human natural killer cells do not inhibit growth of *Cryptococcus neoformans* in the absence of antibody. Infect Immun 58:639-645.

Mitchell TG, Perfect JR. 1995. Cryptococcosis in the era of AIDS--100 years after the discovery of *Cryptococcus neoformans*. Clin Microbiol Rev 8:515-548.

Mody CH, Chen GH, Jackson C, Curtis JL, Toews GB. 1994. In vivo depletion of murine CD8 positive T cells impairs survival during infection with a highly virulent strain of *Cryptococcus neoformans*. Mycopathologia 125:7-17.

Mody CH, Lipscomb MF, Street NE, Toews GB. 1990. Depletion of CD4+ (L3T4+) lymphocytes in vivo impairs murine host defense to *Cryptococcus neoformans*. J Immunol 144:1472-1477.

Montagnoli C, Bozza S, Bacci A, Gaziano R, Mosci P, Morschhauser J, Pitzurra L, Kopf M, Cutler J, Romani L. 2003. A role for antibodies in the generation of memory antifungal immunity. Eur J Immunol 33:1193-1204.

Monteiro da Silva J, Andreotti P, Benard G, Soares C, Miranda E, Mendes-Giannini M. 2007. Epithelial cells treated with genistein inhibit adhesion and endocytosis of *Paracoccidioides brasiliensis*. Antonie Van Leeuwenhoek 92: 129-135.

Moreira AP, Dias-Melicio LA, Soares AM. 2010. Interleukin-10 but not Transforming Growth Factor beta inhibits murine activated macrophages *Paracoccidioides brasiliensis* killing: effect on H2O2 and NO production. Cell Immunol 263:196-203.

Mori S, Levin P. 2009. A brief review of potential mechanisms of immune reconstitution inflammatory syndrome in HIV following antiretroviral therapy. Int J STD AIDS 20:447-452.

Morris A, Sciurba FC, Lebedeva IP, Githaiga A, Elliott WM, Hogg JC, Huang L, Norris KA. 2004. Association of chronic obstructive pulmonary disease severity and *Pneumocystis* colonization. Am J Respir Crit Care Med 170:408-413.

Morris A, Sciurba FC, Norris KA. 2008a. *Pneumocystis*: a novel pathogen in chronic obstructive pulmonary disease? Copd 5:43-51.

Morris A, Wei K, Afshar K, Huang L. 2008b. Epidemiology and clinical significance of *Pneumocystis* colonization. J Infect Dis 197:10-17.

Morrison BE, Park SJ, Mooney JM, Mehrad B. 2003. Chemokine-mediated recruitment of NK cells is a critical host defense mechanism in invasive aspergillosis. J Clin Invest 112:1862-1870.

Mosmann TR, Cherwinski H, Bond MW, Giedlin MA, Coffman RL. 1986. Two types of murine helper T cell clone. I. Definition according to profiles of lymphokine activities and secreted proteins. J Immunol 136:2348-2357.

Mukherjee J, Nussbaum G, Scharff MD, Casadevall A. 1995a. Protective and nonprotective monoclonal antibodies to *Cryptococcus neoformans* originating from one B cell. J Exp Med 181:405-409.

Mukherjee J, Scharff MD, Casadevall A. 1995b. Variable efficacy of passive antibody administration against diverse *Cryptococcus neoformans* strains. Infect Immun 63:3353-3359.

Mukherjee S, Lee SC, Casadevall A. 1995c. Antibodies to *Cryptococcus neoformans* glucuronoxylomannan enhance antifungal activity of murine macrophages. Infect Immun 63:573-579.

Muller U, Stenzel W, Kohler G, Werner C, Polte T, Hansen G, Schutze N, Straubinger RK, Blessing M, McKenzie AN, Brombacher F, Alber G. 2007. IL-13 induces disease-promoting type 2 cytokines, alternatively activated macrophages and allergic inflammation during pulmonary infection of mice with *Cryptococcus neoformans*. J Immunol 179:5367-5377.

Murdoch DM, Venter WD, Feldman C, Van Rie A. 2008. Incidence and risk factors for the immune reconstitution inflammatory syndrome in HIV patients in South Africa: a prospective study. AIDS 22:601-610.

Murphy JW, Hidore MR, Nabavi N. 1991. Binding interactions of murine natural killer cells with the fungal target *Cryptococcus neoformans*. Infect Immun 59:1476-1488.

Murphy JW, McDaniel DO. 1982. In vitro reactivity of natural killer (NK) cells against *Cryptococcus neoformans*. J Immunol 128:1577-1583.

Mylonakis E, Barlam TF, Flanigan T, Rich JD. 1998. Pulmonary aspergillosis and invasive disease in AIDS: review of 342 cases. Chest 114:251-262.

Nabavi N, Murphy JW. 1985. In vitro binding of natural killer cells to *Cryptococcus neoformans* targets. Infect Immun 50:50-57.

Nakamura K, Miyagi K, Koguchi Y, Kinjo Y, Uezu K, Kinjo T, Akamine M, Fujita J, Kawamura I, Mitsuyama M, Adachi Y, Ohno N, Takeda K, Akira S, Miyazato A, Kaku M, Kawakami K. 2006. Limited contribution of Toll-like receptor 2 and 4 to the host response to a fungal infectious pathogen, *Cryptococcus neoformans*. FEMS Immunol Med Microbiol 47:148-154.

Nakamura K, Miyazato A, Xiao G, Hatta M, Inden K, Aoyagi T, Shiratori K, Takeda K, Akira S, Saijo S, Iwakura Y, Adachi Y, Ohno N, Suzuki K, Fujita J, Kaku M, Kawakami K.

2008. Deoxynucleic Acids from *Cryptococcus neoformans* Activate Myeloid Dendritic Cells via a TLR9-Dependent Pathway. J Immunol 180:4067-4074.

Nelson MP, Christmann BS, Werner JL, Metz AE, Trevor JL, Lowell CA, Steele C. 2011. IL-33 and M2a alveolar macrophages promote lung defense against the atypical fungal pathogen *Pneumocystis murina.* J Immunol 186:2372-2381.

Netea MG, Van Der Graaf CA, Vonk AG, Verschueren I, Van Der Meer JW, Kullberg BJ. 2002. The role of toll-like receptor (TLR) 2 and TLR4 in the host defense against disseminated candidiasis. J Infect Dis 185:1483-1489.

Netea MG, Warris A, Van der Meer JW, Fenton MJ, Verver-Janssen TJ, Jacobs LE, Andresen T, Verweij PE, Kullberg BJ. 2003. *Aspergillus fumigatus* evades immune recognition during germination through loss of toll-like receptor-4-mediated signal transduction. J Infect Dis 188:320-326.

Nevez G, Raccurt C, Jounieaux V, Dei-Cas E, Mazars E. 1999. Pneumocystosis versus pulmonary *Pneumocystis carinii* colonization in HIV-negative and HIV-positive patients. AIDS 13:535-536.

Newman KC, Riley EM. 2007. Whatever turns you on: accessory-cell-dependent activation of NK cells by pathogens. Nat Rev Immunol 7:279-291.

Newman S, Chaturvedi S, Klein B. 1995. The WI-1 antigen of *Blastomyces dermatitidis* yeasts mediates binding to human macrophage CD11b/CD18 (CR3) and CD14. J Immunol 154:753-761.

Newman SL, Gootee L, Gabay JE. 1993. Human neutrophil-mediated fungistasis against *Histoplasma capsulatum*. Localization of fungistatic activity to the azurophil granules. Journal Clin Invest 92:624-631.

Newman SL, Gootee L, Kidd C, Ciraolo GM, Morris R. 1997. Activation of human macrophage fungistatic activity against *Histoplasma capsulatum* upon adherence to type 1 collagen matrices. J Immunol 158:1779-1786.

Nooney L, Matthews RC, Burnie JP. 2005. Evaluation of Mycograb, amphotericin B, caspofungin, and fluconazole in combination against *Cryptococcus neoformans* by checkerboard and time-kill methodologies. Diagn Microbiol Infect Dis 51:19-29.

Norris KA, Morris A, Patil S, Fernandes E. 2006. *Pneumocystis* colonization, airway inflammation, and pulmonary function decline in acquired immunodeficiency syndrome. Immunol Res 36:175-187.

Nosanchuk JD, Steenbergen JN, Shi L, Deepe GS, Jr., Casadevall A. 2003. Antibodies to a cell surface histone-like protein protect against *Histoplasma capsulatum*. J Clin Invest 112:1164-1175.

Noverr MC, Cox GM, Perfect JR, Huffnagle GB. 2003. Role of PLB1 in pulmonary inflammation and cryptococcal eicosanoid production. Infect Immun 71:1538-1547.

Nussbaum G, Anandasabapathy S, Mukherjee J, Fan M, Casadevall A, Scharff MD. 1999. Molecular and idiotypic analyses of the antibody response to *Cryptococcus neoformans* glucuronoxylomannan-protein conjugate vaccine in autoimmune and nonautoimmune mice. Infect Immun 67:4469-4476.

Odio CM, Navarrete M, Carrillo JM, Mora L, Carranza A. 1999. Disseminated histoplasmosis in infants. Pediatr Infect Dis J 18:1065-1068.

Olszewski MA, Huffnagle GB, Traynor TR, McDonald RA, Cook DN, Toews GB. 2001. Regulatory effects of macrophage inflammatory protein 1alpha/CCL3 on the development of immunity to *Cryptococcus neoformans* depend on expression of early inflammatory cytokines. Infect Immun 69:6256-6263.

Osterholzer JJ, Curtis JL, Polak T, Ames T, Chen G-H, McDonald R, Huffnagle GB, Toews GB. 2008. CCR2 Mediates Conventional Dendritic Cell Recruitment and the Formation of Bronchovascular Mononuclear Cell Infiltrates in the Lungs of Mice Infected with *Cryptococcus neoformans*. J Immunol 181:610-620.

Osterholzer JJ, Milam JE, Chen GH, Toews GB, Huffnagle GB, Olszewski MA. 2009a. Role of dendritic cells and alveolar macrophages in regulating early host defense against pulmonary infection with *Cryptococcus neoformans*. Infect Immun 77:3749-3758.

Osterholzer JJ, Surana R, Milam JE, Montano GT, Chen GH, Sonstein J, Curtis JL, Huffnagle GB, Toews GB, Olszewski MA. 2009b. Cryptococcal urease promotes the accumulation of immature dendritic cells and a non-protective T2 immune response within the lung. Am J Pathol 174:932-943.

Oykhman P, Mody CH. 2010. Direct microbicidal activity of cytotoxic T-lymphocytes. J Biomed Biotechnol 2010:249482.

Pappas PG, Alexander BD, Andes DR, Hadley S, Kauffman CA, Freifeld A, Anaissie EJ, Brumble LM, Herwaldt L, Ito J, Kontoyiannis DP, Lyon GM, Marr KA, Morrison VA, Park BJ, Patterson TF, Perl TM, Oster RA, Schuster MG, Walker R, Walsh TJ, Wannemuehler KA, Chiller TM. 2010. Invasive fungal infections among organ transplant recipients: results of the Transplant-Associated Infection Surveillance Network (TRANSNET). Clin Infect Dis 50:1101-1111.

Paris S, Boisvieux-Ulrich E, Crestani B, Houcine O, Taramelli D, Lombardi L, Latge JP. 1997. Internalization of *Aspergillus fumigatus* conidia by epithelial and endothelial cells. Infect Immun 65:1510-1514.

Park BJ, Wannemuehler KA, Marston BJ, Govender N, Pappas PG, Chiller TM. 2009. Estimation of the current global burden of cryptococcal meningitis among persons living with HIV/AIDS. AIDS 23:525-530.

Park SJ, Burdick MD, Brix WK, Stoler MH, Askew DS, Strieter RM, Mehrad B. 2010. Neutropenia enhances lung dendritic cell recruitment in response to *Aspergillus* via a cytokine-to-chemokine amplification loop. J Immunol 185:6190-6197.

Patino MM, Williams D, Ahrens J, Graybill JR. 1987. Experimental histoplasmosis in the beige mouse. J Leuk Biol 41:228-235.

Peracoli MT, Fortes MR, Da Silva MF, Montenegro MR. 1995. Natural killer cell activity in experimental paracoccidioidomycosis of the Syrian hamster. Rev Inst Med Trop Sao Paulo 37:129-136.

Perfect JR, Casadevall A. 2002. Cryptococcosis. Infect Dis Clin N Am 16:837-874.

Petkus AF, Baum LL. 1987. Natural killer cell inhibition of young spherules and endospores of *Coccidioides immitis*. J Immunol 139:3107-3111.

Pinzan CF, Ruas LP, Casabona-Fortunato AS, Carvalho FC, Roque-Barreira MC. 2010. Immunological basis for the gender differences in murine *Paracoccidioides brasiliensis* infection. PLoS One 5:e10757.

Pirofski LA. 2001. Polysaccharides, mimotopes and vaccines for fungal and encapsulated pathogens. Trends Microbiol 9:445-451.

Rachini A, Pietrella D, Lupo P, Torosantucci A, Chiani P, Bromuro C, Proietti C, Bistoni F, Cassone A, Vecchiarelli A. 2007. An anti-beta-glucan monoclonal antibody inhibits growth and capsule formation of *Cryptococcus neoformans* in vitro and exerts therapeutic, anticryptococcal activity in vivo. Infect Immun 75:5085-5094.

Ramaprakash H, Ito T, Standiford TJ, Kunkel SL, Hogaboam CM. 2009. Toll-like receptor 9 modulates immune responses to *Aspergillus fumigatus* conidia in immunodeficient and allergic mice. Infect Immun 77:108-119.

Ramirez-Ortiz ZG, Lee CK, Wang JP, Boon L, Specht CA, Levitz SM. 2011. A Nonredundant Role for Plasmacytoid Dendritic Cells in Host Defense against the Human Fungal Pathogen *Aspergillus fumigatus*. Cell Host Microbe 9:415-424.

Ramirez-Ortiz ZG, Specht CA, Wang JP, Lee CK, Bartholomeu DC, Gazzinelli RT, Levitz SM. 2008. Toll-like receptor 9-dependent immune activation by unmethylated CpG motifs in *Aspergillus fumigatus* DNA. Infect Immun 76:2123-2129.

Rayhane N, Lortholary O, Fitting C, Callebert J, Huerre M, Dromer F, Cavaillon JM. 1999. Enhanced sensitivity of tumor necrosis factor/lymphotoxin-alpha-deficient mice to *Cryptococcus neoformans* infection despite increased levels of nitrite/nitrate, interferon-gamma, and interleukin-12. J Infect Dis 180:1637-1647.

Retini C, Vecchiarelli A, Monari C, Tascini C, Bistoni F, Kozel TR. 1996. Capsular polysaccharide of *Cryptococcus neoformans* induces proinflammatory cytokine release by human neutrophils. Infect Immun 64:2897-2903.

Rivera J, Casadevall A. 2005. Mouse genetic background is a major determinant of isotype-related differences for antibody-mediated protective efficacy against *Cryptococcus neoformans*. J Immunol 174:8017-8026.

Rivera J, Mukherjee J, Weiss LM, Casadevall A. 2002. Antibody efficacy in murine pulmonary *Cryptococcus neoformans* infection: a role for nitric oxide. J Immunol 168:3419-3427.

Rodrigues ML, Shi L, Barreto-Bergter E, Nimrichter L, Farias SE, Rodrigues EG, Travassos LR, Nosanchuk JD. 2007. Monoclonal antibody to fungal glucosylceramide protects mice against lethal *Cryptococcus neoformans* infection. Clin Vaccine Immunol 14:1372-1376.

Romani L, Mencacci A, Tonnetti L, Spaccapelo R, Cenci E, Puccetti P, Wolf SF, Bistoni F. 1994. IL-12 is both required and prognostic in vivo for T helper type 1 differentiation in murine candidiasis. J Immunol 153:5167-5175.

Romani L, Puccetti P. 2008. Immune regulation and tolerance to fungi in the lungs and skin. Chem Immunol Allergy 94:124-137.

Rosas AL, Nosanchuk JD, Casadevall A. 2001. Passive immunization with melanin-binding monoclonal antibodies prolongs survival of mice with lethal *Cryptococcus neoformans* infection. Infect Immun 69:3410-3412.

Ruas LP, Bernardes ES, Fermino ML, de Oliveira LL, Hsu DK, Liu FT, Chammas R, Roque-Barreira MC. 2009. Lack of galectin-3 drives response to *Paracoccidioides brasiliensis* toward a Th2-biased immunity. PLoS One 4:e4519.

Rudner XL, Happel KI, Young EA, Shellito JE. 2007. Interleukin-23 (IL-23)-IL-17 cytokine axis in murine *Pneumocystis carinii* infection. Infect Immun 75:3055-3061.

Salkowski CA, Balish E. 1991. Role of natural killer cells in resistance to systemic cryptococcosis. J Leuk Biol 50:151-159.

Savage DC, Madin SH. 1968. Cellular responses in lungs of immunized mice to intranasal infection with *Coccidioides immitis*. Sabouraudia 6:94-102.

Scheckelhoff M, Deepe GS, Jr. 2005. A deficiency in gamma interferon or interleukin-10 modulates T-Cell-dependent responses to heat shock protein 60 from *Histoplasma capsulatum*. Infect Immun 73:2129-2134.

Schmidt S, Tramsen L, Hanisch M, Latge JP, Huenecke S, Koehl U, Lehrnbecher T. 2011. Human natural killer cells exhibit direct activity against *Aspergillus fumigatus* hyphae, but not against resting conidia. J Infect Dis 203:430-435.

Schrettl M, Ibrahim-Granet O, Droin S, Huerre M, Latge JP, Haas H. 2010. The crucial role of the *Aspergillus fumigatus* siderophore system in interaction with alveolar macrophages. Microbes Infect 12:1035-1041.

Seddiki N, Sasson SC, Santner-Nanan B, Munier M, van Bockel D, Ip S, Marriott D, Pett S, Nanan R, Cooper DA, Zaunders JJ, Kelleher AD. 2009. Proliferation of weakly suppressive regulatory CD4+ T cells is associated with over-active CD4+ T-cell responses in HIV-positive patients with mycobacterial immune restoration disease. Eur J Immunol 39:391-403.

Serrano-Gomez D, Dominguez-Soto A, Ancochea J, Jimenez-Heffernan JA, Leal JA, Corbi AL. 2004. Dendritic cell-specific intercellular adhesion molecule 3-grabbing nonintegrin mediates binding and internalization of *Aspergillus fumigatus* conidia by dendritic cells and macrophages. J Immunol 173:5635-5643.

Shankar EM, Vignesh R, Velu V, Murugavel KG, Sekar R, Balakrishnan P, Lloyd CA, Saravanan S, Solomon S, Kumarasamy N. 2008. Does CD4+CD25+foxp3+ cell (Treg) and IL-10 profile determine susceptibility to immune reconstitution inflammatory syndrome (IRIS) in HIV disease? J Inflamm (Lond) 5:2.

Shellito JE, Tate C, Ruan S, Kolls J. 2000. Murine CD4+ T lymphocyte subsets and host defense against *Pneumocystis carinii*. J Infect Dis 181:2011-2017.

Shoham S, Levitz SM. 2005. The immune response to fungal infections. Br J Haematol 129:569-582.

Shubitz LF, Yu JJ, Hung CY, Kirkland TN, Peng T, Perrill R, Simons J, Xue J, Herr RA, Cole GT, Galgiani JN. 2006. Improved protection of mice against lethal respiratory infection with *Coccidioides posadasii* using two recombinant antigens expressed as a single protein. Vaccine 24:5904-5911.

Silva AJ, Benitez JA. 2005. Th1-type immune response to a *Coccidioides immitis* antigen delivered by an attenuated strain of the non-invasive enteropathogen Vibrio cholerae. FEMS Immunol Med Microbiol 43:393-398.

Silva MFd, Napimoga MH, Rodrigues DBR, Pereira SAL, Silva CL. 2011. Phenotypic and functional characterization of pulmonary macrophages subpopulations after intratracheal injection of *Paracoccidioides brasiliensis* cell wall components. Immunobiol 216:821-831.

Silvana dos Santos S, Ferreira KS, Almeida SR. 2011. *Paracoccidioides brasilinsis*-Induced Migration of Dendritic Cells and Subsequent T-Cell Activation in the Lung-Draining Lymph Nodes. PLoS ONE 6:e19690.

Singh N, Gayowski T, Wagener MM, Marino IR. 1997. Clinical spectrum of invasive cryptococcosis in liver transplant recipients receiving tacrolimus. Clin Transplant 11:66-70.

Singh N, Lortholary O, Alexander BD, Gupta KL, John GT, Pursell K, Munoz P, Klintmalm GB, Stosor V, del Busto R, Limaye AP, Somani J, Lyon M, Houston S, House AA, Pruett TL, Orloff S, Humar A, Dowdy L, Garcia-Diaz J, Kalil AC, Fisher RA, Husain

S. 2005. An immune reconstitution syndrome-like illness associated with *Cryptococcus neoformans* infection in organ transplant recipients. Clin Infect Dis 40:1756-1761.

Singh N, Perfect JR. 2007. Immune reconstitution syndrome associated with opportunistic mycoses. Lancet Infect Dis 7:395-401.

Soares DA, de Andrade RV, Silva SS, Bocca AL, Soares Felipe SM, Petrofeza S. 2010. Extracellular *Paracoccidioides brasiliensis* phospholipase B involvement in alveolar macrophage interaction. BMC Microbiol 10:241.

Soroosh P, Doherty TA. 2009. Th9 and allergic disease. Immunology 127:450-458.

Spitzer ED, Spitzer SG, Freundlich LF, Casadevall A. 1993. Persistence of initial infection in recurrent *Cryptococcus neoformans* meningitis. Lancet 341:595-596.

Steele C, Zheng M, Young E, Marrero L, Shellito JE, Kolls JK. 2002. Increased host resistance against *Pneumocystis carinii* pneumonia in gammadelta T-cell-deficient mice: protective role of gamma interferon and CD8(+) T cells. Infect Immun 70:5208-5215.

Stevens TL, Bossie A, Sanders VM, Fernandez-Botran R, Coffman RL, Mosmann TR, Vitetta ES. 1988. Regulation of antibody isotype secretion by subsets of antigen-specific helper T cells. Nature 334:255-258.

Strasser JE, Newman SL, Ciraolo GM, Morris RE, Howell ML, Dean GE. 1999. Regulation of the macrophage vacuolar ATPase and phagosome-lysosome fusion by *Histoplasma capsulatum*. J Immunol 162:6148-6154.

Suchyta MR, Smith JG, Graybill JR. 1988. The role of natural killer cells in histoplasmosis. Am Rev Resp Dis 138:578-582.

Syme RM, Spurrell JCL, Amankwah EK, Green FHY, Mody CH. 2002. Primary dendritic cells phagocytose *Cryptococcus neoformans* via mannose receptors and Fc gamma receptor II for presentation to T lymphocytes. Infect Immun 70:5972-5981.

Tarcha EJ, Basrur V, Hung CY, Gardner MJ, Cole GT. 2006. A recombinant aspartyl protease of *Coccidioides posadasii* induces protection against pulmonary coccidioidomycosis in mice. Infect Immun 74:516-527.

Taylor PR, Brown GD, Reid DM, Willment JA, Martinez-Pomares L, Gordon S, Wong SYC. 2002. The β-Glucan Receptor, Dectin-1, Is Predominantly Expressed on the Surface of Cells of the Monocyte/Macrophage and Neutrophil Lineages. J Immunol 169:3876-3882.

Taylor PR, Tsoni SV, Willment JA, Dennehy KM, Rosas M, Findon H, Haynes K, Steele C, Botto M, Gordon S, Brown GD. 2007. Dectin-1 is required for beta-glucan recognition and control of fungal infection. Nat Immunol 8:31-38.

Torosantucci A, Bromuro C, Chiani P, De Bernardis F, Berti F, Galli C, Norelli F, Bellucci C, Polonelli L, Costantino P, Rappuoli R, Cassone A. 2005. A novel glyco-conjugate vaccine against fungal pathogens. J Exp Med 202:597-606.

Traynor TR, Kuziel WA, Toews GB, Huffnagle GB. 2000. CCR2 Expression Determines T1 Versus T2 Polarization During Pulmonary *Cryptococcus neoformans* Infection. J Immunol 164:2021-2027.

Tucker SC, Casadevall A. 2002. Replication of *Cryptococcus neoformans* in macrophages is accompanied by phagosomal permeabilization and accumulation of vesicles containing polysaccharide in the cytoplasm. Proc Natl Acad Sci USA 99:3165-3170.

Uezu K, Kawakami K, Miyagi K, Kinjo Y, Kinjo T, Ishikawa H, Saito A. 2004. Accumulation of gammadelta T cells in the lungs and their regulatory roles in Th1 response and host defense against pulmonary infection with *Cryptococcus neoformans*. J Immunol 172:7629-7634.

Voelz K, Lammas DA, May RC. 2009. Cytokine signaling regulates the outcome of intracellular macrophage parasitism by *Cryptococcus neoformans*. Infect Immun.

Wang J, Gigliotti F, Bhagwat SP, Maggirwar SB, Wright TW. 2007. Pneumocystis stimulates MCP-1 production by alveolar epithelial cells through a JNK-dependent mechanism. Am J Phys Lung Cell Mol Phys 292:L1495-1505.

Wang J, Gigliotti F, Maggirwar S, Johnston C, Finkelstein JN, Wright TW. 2005. *Pneumocystis carinii* activates the NF-kappaB signaling pathway in alveolar epithelial cells. Infect Immun 73:2766-2777.

Wang JE, Warris A, Ellingsen EA, Jorgensen PF, Flo TH, Espevik T, Solberg R, Verweij PE, Aasen AO. 2001. Involvement of CD14 and toll-like receptors in activation of human monocytes by *Aspergillus fumigatus* hyphae. Infect Immun 69:2402-2406.

Warschkau H, Yu H, Kiderlen AF. 1998. Activation and suppression of natural cellular immune functions by *Pneumocystis carinii*. Immunobiol 198:343-360.

Wegner TN, Reed RE, Trautman RJ, Beavers CD. 1972. Some evidence for the development of a phagocytic response by polymorphonuclear leukocytes recovered from the venous blood of dogs inoculated with *Coccidioides immitis* or vaccinated with an irradiated spherule vaccine. Am Rev Resp Dis 105:845-849.

Winters MS, Chan Q, Caruso JA, Deepe GS, Jr. 2010. Metallomic analysis of macrophages infected with *Histoplasma capsulatum* reveals a fundamental role for zinc in host defenses. J Infect Dis 202:1136-1145.

Wormley FL, Jr., Perfect JR, Steele C, Cox GM. 2007. Protection Against Cryptococcosis using a Murine Interferon-gamma Producing *Cryptococcus neoformans* Strain. Infect Immun 75:1453-1462.

Wozniak KL, Hardison SE, Kolls JK, Wormley FL. 2011a. Role of IL-17A on resolution of pulmonary *C. neoformans* infection. PLoS One 6:e17204.

Wozniak KL, Levitz SM. 2008. *Cryptococcus neoformans* enters the endolysosomal pathway of dendritic cells and is killed by lysosomal components. Infect Immun 76:4764-4771.

Wozniak KL, Ravi S, Macias S, Young ML, Olszewski MA, Steele C, Wormley FL. 2009. Insights into the mechanisms of protective immunity against *Cryptococcus neoformans* infection using a mouse model of pulmonary cryptococcosis. PLoS ONE 4:e6854.

Wozniak KL, Vyas JM, Levitz SM. 2006. In Vivo Role of Dendritic Cells in a Murine Model of Pulmonary Cryptococcosis. Infect Immun 74:3817-3824.

Wozniak KL, Young ML, Wormley FL, Jr. 2011b. Protective immunity against experimental pulmonary cryptococcosis in T cell-depleted mice. Clin Vaccine Immunol 18:717-723.

Wu-Hsieh B, Howard DH. 1984. Inhibition of growth of *Histoplasma capsulatum* by lymphokine-stimulated macrophages. J Immunol 132:2593-2597.

Wu-Hsieh B, Zlotnik A, Howard DH. 1984. T-cell hybridoma-produced lymphokine that activates macrophages to suppress intracellular growth of Histoplasma capsulatum. Infect Immun 43:380-385.

Wuthrich M, Filutowicz HI, Klein BS. 2000. Mutation of the WI-1 gene yields an attenuated *Blastomyces dermatitidis* strain that induces host resistance. J Clin Invest 106:1381-1389.

Wuthrich M, Filutowicz HI, Warner T, Deepe GS, Jr., Klein BS. 2003. Vaccine immunity to pathogenic fungi overcomes the requirement for CD4 help in exogenous antigen presentation to CD8+ T cells: implications for vaccine development in immune-deficient hosts. J Exp Med 197:1405-1416.

Wuthrich M, Filutowicz HI, Warner T, Klein BS. 2002. Requisite elements in vaccine immunity to *Blastomyces dermatitidis*: plasticity uncovers vaccine potential in immune-deficient hosts. J Immunol 169:6969-6976.

Wuthrich M, Fisette PL, Filutowicz HI, Klein BS. 2006. Differential requirements of T cell subsets for CD40 costimulation in immunity to *Blastomyces dermatitidis*. J Immunol 176:5538-5547.

Wuthrich M, Gern B, Hung CY, Ersland K, Rocco N, Pick-Jacobs J, Galles K, Filutowicz H, Warner T, Evans M, Cole G, Klein B. 2011. Vaccine-induced protection against 3 systemic mycoses endemic to North America requires Th17 cells in mice. J Clin Invest 121:554-568.

Wuthrich M, Warner T, Klein BS. 2005. IL-12 is required for induction but not maintenance of protective, memory responses to *Blastomyces dermatitidis*: implications for vaccine development in immune-deficient hosts. J Immunol 175:5288-5297.

Xue J, Chen X, Selby D, Hung CY, Yu JJ, Cole GT. 2009. A genetically engineered live attenuated vaccine of *Coccidioides posadasii* protects BALB/c mice against coccidioidomycosis. Infect Immun 77:3196-3208.

Yoneda K, Walzer PD. 1980. Interaction of *Pneumocystis carinii* with host lungs: an ultrastructural study. Infect Immun 29:692-703.

Young M, Macias S, Thomas D, Wormley FL, Jr. 2009. A proteomic-based approach for the identification of immunodominant *Cryptococcus neoformans* proteins. Proteomics 9:2578-2588.

Yu ML, Limper AH. 1997. *Pneumocystis carinii* induces ICAM-1 expression in lung epithelial cells through a TNF-alpha-mediated mechanism. Am J Physiol 273:L1103-1111.

Yuan R, Casadevall A, Spira G, Scharff MD. 1995. Isotype switching from IgG3 to IgG1 converts a nonprotective murine antibody to *Cryptococcus neoformans* into a protective antibody. J Immunol 154:1810-1816.

Yuan RR, Casadevall A, Oh J, Scharff MD. 1997. T cells cooperate with passive antibody to modify *Cryptococcus neoformans* infection in mice. Proc Natl Acad Sci USA 94:2483-2488.

Yuan RR, Clynes R, Oh J, Ravetch JV, Scharff MD. 1998a. Antibody-mediated modulation of *Cryptococcus neoformans* infections is dependent on distinct Fc receptor functions and IgG subclasses. J Exp Med 187:641-648.

Yuan RR, Spira G, Oh J, Paizi M, Casadevall A, Scharff MD. 1998b. Isotype switching increases efficacy of antibody protection against *Cryptococcus neoformans* infection in mice. Infect Immun 66:1057-1062.

Zaragoza O, Casadevall A. 2004. Antibodies produced in response to *Cryptococcus neoformans* pulmonary infection in mice have characteristics of nonprotective antibodies. Infect Immun 72:4271-4274.

Zaragoza O, Rodrigues ML, De Jesus M, Frases S, Dadachova E, Casadevall A. 2009. The capsule of the fungal pathogen *Cryptococcus neoformans*. Adv Appl Microbiol 68:133-216.

Zelante T, De Luca A, Bonifazi P, Montagnoli C, Bozza S, Moretti S, Belladonna ML, Vacca C, Conte C, Mosci P, Bistoni F, Puccetti P, Kastelein RA, Kopf M, Romani L. 2007. IL-23 and the Th17 pathway promote inflammation and impair antifungal immune resistance. Eur J Immunol 37:2695-2706.

Zhang H, Zhong Z, Pirofski LA. 1997. Peptide epitopes recognized by a human anti-cryptococcal glucuronoxylomannan antibody. Infect Immun 65:1158-1164.

Zhang Y, Wang F, Tompkins KC, McNamara A, Jain AV, Moore BB, Toews GB, Huffnagle GB, Olszewski MA. 2009. Robust Th1 and Th17 immunity supports pulmonary clearance but cannot prevent systemic dissemination of highly virulent *Cryptococcus neoformans* H99. Am J Pathol 175:2489-2500.

Zhang Z, Liu R, Noordhoek JA, Kauffman HF. 2005. Interaction of airway epithelial cells (A549) with spores and mycelium of *Aspergillus fumigatus*. J Infect 51:375-382.

Zheng CF, Jones GJ, Shi M, Wiseman JC, Marr KJ, Berenger BM, Huston SM, Gill MJ, Krensky AM, Kubes P, Mody CH. 2008. Late expression of granulysin by microbicidal CD4+ T cells requires PI3K- and STAT5-dependent expression of IL-2Rbeta that is defective in HIV-infected patients. J Immunol 180:7221-7229.

Zheng CF, Ma LL, Jones GJ, Gill MJ, Krensky AM, Kubes P, Mody CH. 2007. Cytotoxic CD4+ T cells use granulysin to kill *Cryptococcus neoformans*, and activation of this pathway is defective in HIV patients. Blood 109:2049-2057.

Zhong Z, Pirofski LA. 1996. Opsonization of *Cryptococcus neoformans* by human anticryptococcal glucuronoxylomannan antibodies. Infect Immun 64:3446-3450.

Zhong Z, Pirofski LA. 1998. Antifungal activity of a human antiglucuronoxylomannan antibody. Clin Diagn Lab Immunol 5:58-64.

Zhou P, Freidag BL, Caldwell CC, Seder RA. 2001. Perforin is required for primary immunity to *Histoplasma capsulatum*. Journal of immunology 166:1968-1974.

Zhou P, Miller G, Seder RA. 1998. Factors involved in regulating primary and secondary immunity to infection with *Histoplasma capsulatum*: TNF-alpha plays a critical role in maintaining secondary immunity in the absence of IFN-gamma. J Immunol 160:1359-1368.

Zhou P, Sieve MC, Bennett J, Kwon-Chung KJ, Tewari RP, Gazzinelli RT, Sher A, Seder RA. 1995. IL-12 prevents mortality in mice infected with *Histoplasma capsulatum* through induction of IFN-gamma. J Immunol 155:785-795.